Penguin Handbooks

A Baby in the Family

KV-203-564

James and Joyce Robertson have been together as husband and wife, and colleagues, for more than forty years. Their approach to child development reflects much experience of young children, coupled with a deep conviction of the competence of ordinary parents to meet their children's needs. As a young married couple of working-class origins, he from Scotland and she from London, they worked together in the Hampstead Wartime Nurseries run by Anna Freud and Dorothy Burlingham.

After staying at home for twelve years to look after their two daughters, Joyce was for the next eight years attached to a Well Baby Clinic. There she worked with mothers and very young children, and published a number of papers on mother–infant interaction and the influence of early experience upon development. She was also consultant to a residential nursery where she studied the adverse effects of that form of care on infants and young children.

James Robertson is a psychiatric social worker and psychoanalyst. As a research worker in the National Health Service he became deeply concerned about the plight of children in hospitals who, thirty years ago, were allowed little contact with their parents. He made two films, *A Two-Year Old Goes to Hospital* (1952) and *Going to Hospital with Mother* (1958). These two films and a book, *Young Children in Hospital* (1958), are acknowledged to have been a strong influence upon the Platt Report, 1959, on which Ministry of Health policy is based.

In 1965 the Robertsons teamed up within the Tavistock Institute of Human Relations in order to pursue their research into child development. Out of this study, *Young Children in Brief Separation*, came five complementary films which have been widely acclaimed and are an integral part of the teaching of child development in many parts of the world. The Robertsons have travelled widely to lecture and to conduct conferences on their approach to child care. They now run the Robertson Centre whose purpose is 'to promote understanding of the emotional needs of infants and young children'.

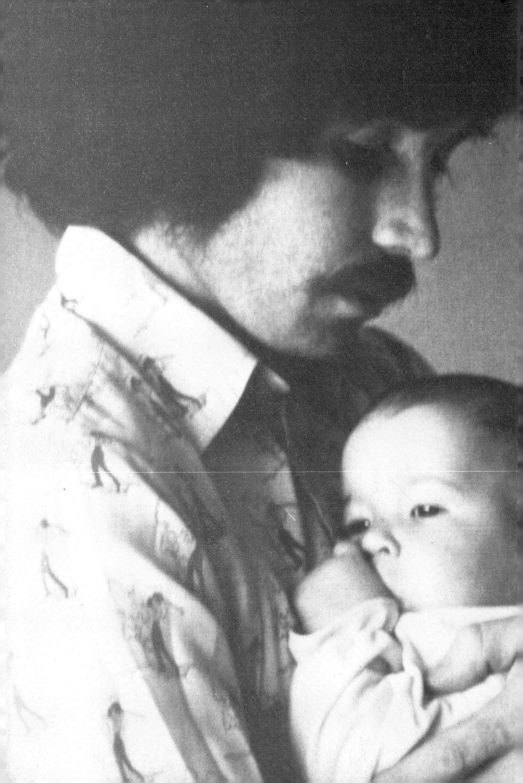

James and Joyce Robertson

A BABY IN THE FAMILY

Loving and Being Loved

Penguin Books

Penguin Books Ltd, Harmondsworth, Middlesex, England
Penguin Books, 625 Madison Avenue, New York, New York 10022, U.S.A.
Penguin Books Australia Ltd, Ringwood, Victoria, Australia
Penguin Books Canada Ltd, 2801 John Street, Markham, Ontario, Canada L3R 1B4
Penguin Books (N.Z.) Ltd, 182–190 Wairau Road, Auckland 10, New Zealand

First published 1982

Composition in Photina by Filmtype Services Limited, Scarborough, North Yorkshire
Printed in Great Britain

Designed by David Grogan

Photographs by James Robertson
with help from the rest of the family

To our grandchildren
PAUL and SARAH

To their mothers
who are our daughters
KATHERINE and JEAN

And to their fathers
FRANK and JOHN

Contents

Foreword

This book is not about mumps and measles, spots and tantrums, nor about milestones of development. It is about loving and being loved.

We hope it will help parents-to-be, especially first-time parents, to know what to expect in the first year of a baby's life, to enjoy the baby more through greater understanding of what goes on between them, and to trust to their own feelings in the care and protection of their baby – by taking a stand, if required, against unnecessary restrictions sometimes met in maternity units, paediatric wards, and elsewhere in child care.

We draw upon those experiences of our two grandchildren Paul and Sarah and their parents which are common to most ordinary families.

The book's emphasis on the importance of early relationships has implications for the professions dealing with young children and their families, and we trust it will be found helpful for teaching about family relationships and emotional development in the first year.

In following the convention of referring to a baby as 'he' we mean of course 'he' or 'she' as appropriate.

We are indebted to The Irving Harris Foundation of Chicago for their support of the study.

London 1981   James Robertson
                                                      Joyce Robertson

Introduction

This book is about ordinary families and the very special babies that are found in them. Despite what is sometimes said about the frequency of family breakdown and about uncaring parents, the great majority of parents are devoted to their children and give them love and security – but they do not make the headlines.

Stand in an infants' school playground as the day finishes and see the heart-warming picture of young mothers with babies in prams, waiting for their 5-year-olds to run out clutching the day's work to show their Mum. These 5-year-olds spill out the trials and tribulations of the school day, and the achievements, knowing they will get sympathy, praise and affection interlaced with the odd rebuke. They know that their Mum (and their Dad) will be protective and loving, interested in the detail of their experiences.

Parents may sometimes long for more freedom, more peace, more sleep; but the children remain the mainspring of their lives. We enjoy them, marvel at them, worry over them and get cross with them. Family life can be tough and tedious, incredibly sweet and marvellous in varying mixtures. But despite its stresses and strains the family is where most of us grow up, and in its richness is still the best environment in which to rear children.

In order to see what is likely to give a good beginning to a family we shall start with the birth of a first baby and follow through to the end of the first year. During that year two people become mother and father, and the baby comes to know he is part of a family. We shall follow the baby as he gradually makes relationships with his parents and grandparents, and as he moves from oneness with his mother to become a separate person.

At first the parents are his whole world. The first playthings are his mother's fingers and face; his muscles strengthen by play on his father's knee; his babbling increases as the parents listen and talk to him. As he reaches to the world beyond them they will be there to facilitate his searching. His curiosity will be keen, his pleasures enhanced by the parents sharing his discoveries.

Then the parents, if things have started reasonably well, will find themselves doing naturally what the baby needs – not all of the time, but most of the time. And as they see the baby flourishing under their care, as he or she becomes more special and more dear to them, they will feel more sure of themselves and ever more deeply committed to him, despite anxiety and tiredness and restrictions of activities.

The more parents enjoy their children and feel them to be special, the more likely the children are to grow into independent adults capable of loving and being loved and of rearing their own children in a similar way.

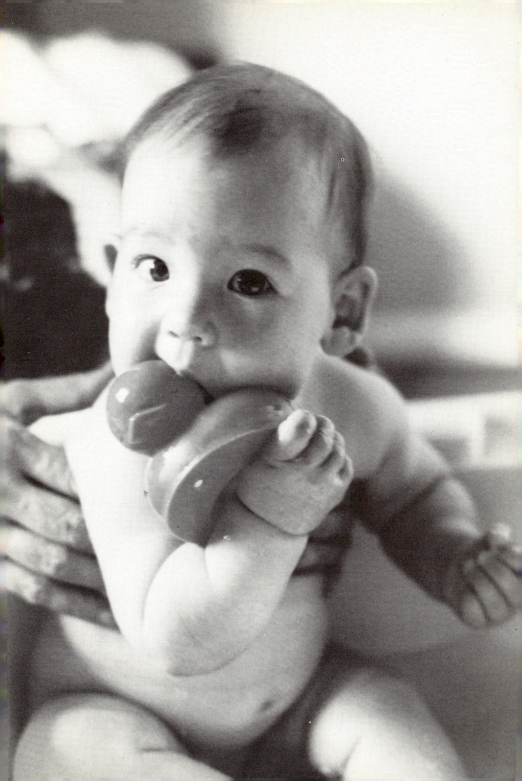

Chapter One

The Love of Parents for their Baby

(Sometimes called 'Bonding')

The special love that most parents feel for their children usually begins at birth and becomes an irresistible commitment to the baby's well-being which deepens as the months go by.

This 'bonding' of parents to their children combines love, concern, protectiveness, pride and pleasure. These override the inevitable irritations and restrictions.

The child whose parents love him in this way is always sure of someone on his side against the world, who is unlikely to abuse or abandon him.

The only true basis for the relationship of a child to mother and father, to other children, and eventually to society, is the first successful relationship between the mother and baby.[1]

D.W. Winnicott

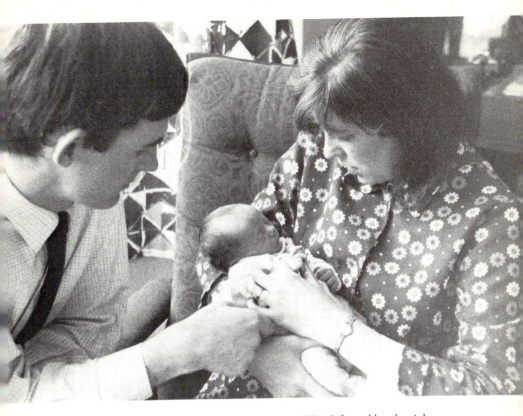

BABY PAUL is 2 days old and weighs just 6lbs. He is the centre of his parents' attention. Katherine and Frank look and touch and talk to him as he sleeps. There is anxiety and tension in the face of the young mother.

The high level of anxiety commonly felt by young mothers can be uncomfortable and sometimes frightening.

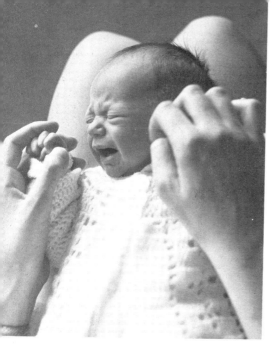

2 weeks

When the baby is unhappy the mother has the satisfaction of restoring him to comfort.

At the breast, Paul seeks eye-to-eye contact ...

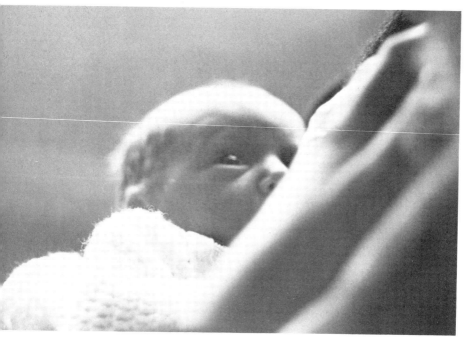

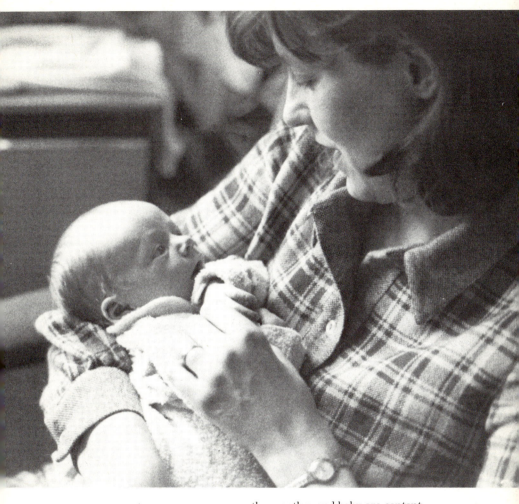

...then mother and baby are content
to look at each other and 'talk'.

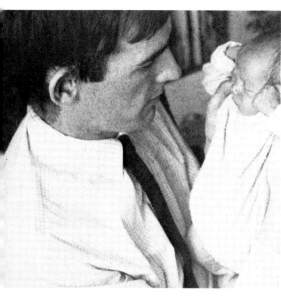

2 weeks

The father takes a closer look. He hasn't had much to do with babies.

He quickly learns that the head is loose.

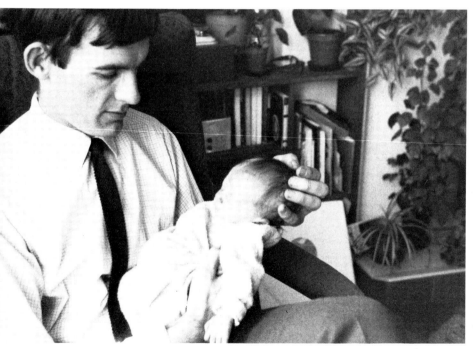

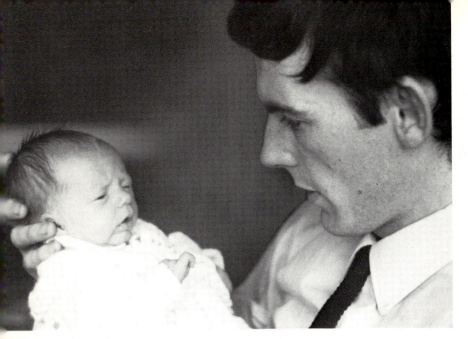

3 weeks

Sometimes father is faced by an unhappy baby. He is concerned and uncertain what to do.

He is pleased when he manages to make the baby comfortable.

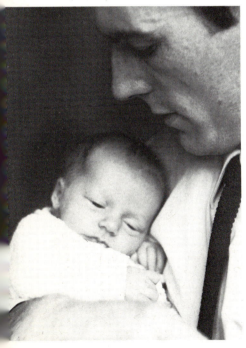

This kind of experience draws father ever closer to his son.

19

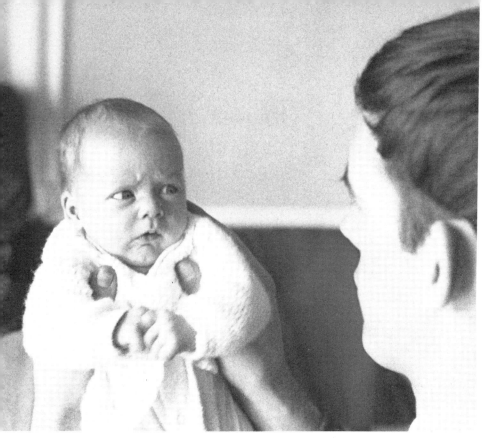

Paul is 5 weeks old. He is used to his mother's voice and touch and smell. But he sees less of his father.

Fathers differ in their attitude to the new-born baby. Some try to keep a distance for the first few weeks, when the baby seems little more than a demanding object that needs fuelling at one end and cleaning at the other. Their interest perks up when the baby begins to smile and gurgle, and becomes easier to hold.

The earlier the father handles his baby, the more deeply he will feel for him. The closer he becomes, the more he will enjoy the baby and be able to tolerate

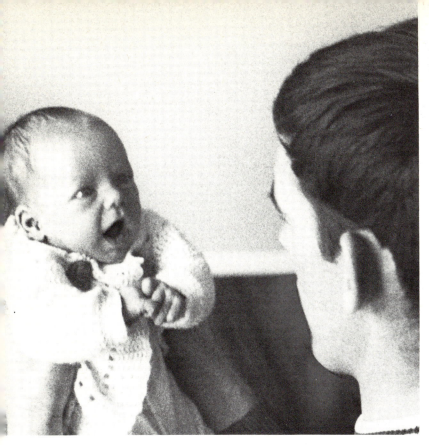

The father gives Paul time to
respond, and is rewarded by a smile.
Another pull on father towards the baby.

the restrictions that a new baby makes on the family. If he can have a week
or two off work at the time of the birth this gives a good start.

But fathers do not have the exceptionally high level of anxiety which for
several weeks after the birth makes the mother specially sensitive to the
baby's needs and draws her close to him.

In ordinary families where father is out all day the mother remains closer
to the baby throughout the first year, with father the best substitute for her.

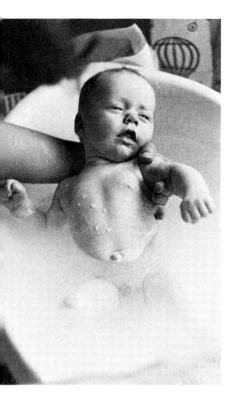
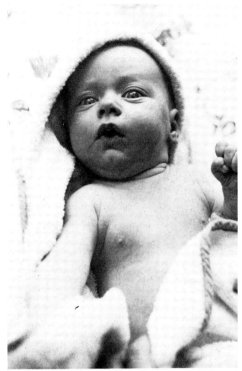

2 months

As she tends her baby throughout
the day, the mother is open to the
appeal of a small being who is totally
dependent upon her. He is helpless,
cuddly, and holds her with an
intense gaze.

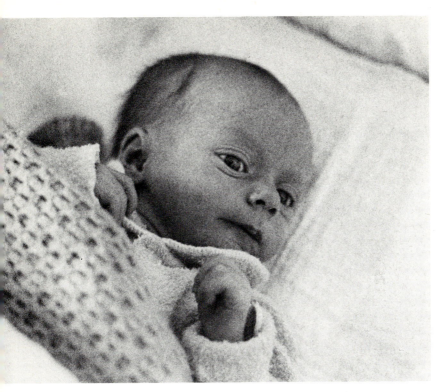

Paul is fed, bathed, warmly wrapped up, and ready for sleep.

Repeated experience of being important to her baby, of being the one who knows him best and who keeps him safe, who can make him comfortable and elicit smiles of pleasure, deepens the feelings of the mother for her baby.

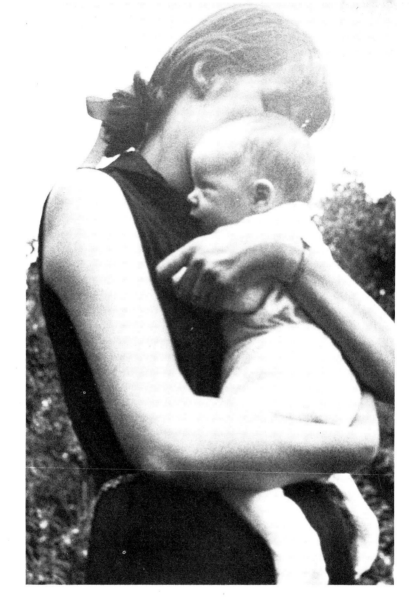

By three months the mother has passed through the early period of heightened anxiety. She is now more confident. She has found by trial and error what comforts him most.

The baby is held close, so that as much of him touches her as is possible. She rocks him and talks to him. She now enjoys Paul in a more serene way.

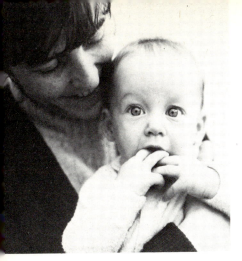

5 months

The mother is pleased by the friendly attention that Paul attracts.

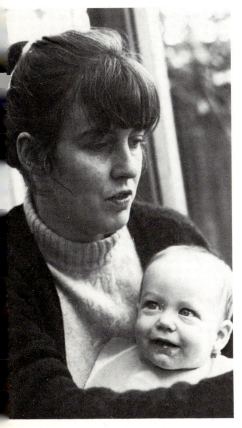

He is interested in what is going on, but still from the safety of his mother's arms. Her encircling arm is symbolically a barrier between the baby and the outside world.

Children are Special to Their Own Parents

'Children are like toothbrushes. They are all much alike, but we prefer our own.' Thus spoke a father.

Most parents see their own children through rose-tinted spectacles. They find them more attractive and more cute than other people's children. This enables them to tolerate their children's less desirable traits (their wakefulness at night, their demands, their sticky fingers) with surprising patience for most, if not all, of the time.

This was true of Paul's parents. Having a baby dependent on them, who responded to them in appealing ways, elicited feelings of protectiveness and affection which could override occasional irritation and constant tiredness. This is the irrational love on which babies thrive and families hold together.

But the baby whose care is shared with an au pair, child minder, or day nursery cannot come to be so 'special' to the mother for the simple reason that she does not have the full experience of meeting his needs, getting his affection, and interacting with him throughout the day. She is likely to be less in tune with her baby, and less tolerant of his behaviour than the mother who is the sole caretaker.

The division of care between the mother and another (or others), and the discontinuity of interaction between mother and baby, must impair her empathy for him and lower his expectations of her. Likewise a father who is little involved with his baby will find him less 'special' than does the father who is much involved.

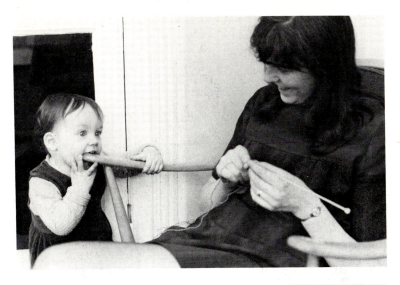

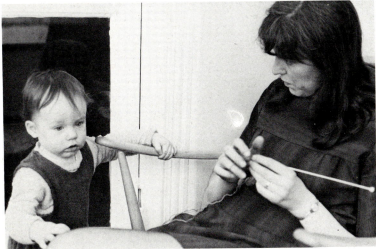

At 11 months Paul finds pleasure in biting on the arm of a chair, and mother stops knitting to enjoy the experience with him.

Then when he hurts his mouth she stops again, and her expression changes to match his. She is now sharing his hurt.

In addition to the protectiveness and the pleasure something else is developing in the mother. There is empathy: she shares his feelings.

At the end of the first year.

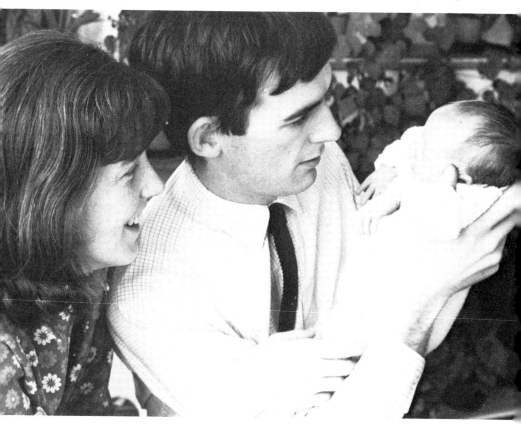

A year ago Katherine and Frank did
not know themselves as father and
mother; they did not know the baby,
and the baby did not know them.

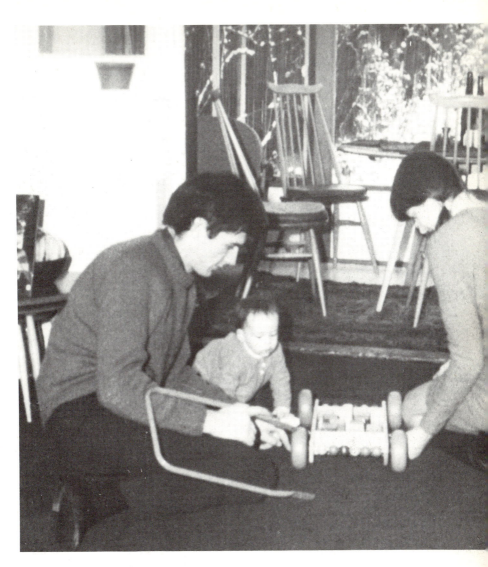

Now, after the ups and downs of the first year, Paul is very special to them. What is important to him matters to them; they are as interested as he is in the new toy. They put his needs before their own pleasures and wishes (not without a grumble sometimes). To the onlooker this may seem excessive indulgence, but to the parents it feels natural and right.

A Closer Look at How Bonding Begins

The bonding of parents to their baby is crucial for the well-being of the whole family. It is fostered or hindered by what happens in the hospital and during the first few weeks at home.

This section looks more closely at the early weeks when bonding begins. The subjects are our second grandchild, Sarah, and her parents, John and Jean. Sarah was born full-term, healthy, 9lbs in weight. John was with Jean throughout a lengthy labour, but not for the birth.

In the labour ward and delivery room they were well supported by considerate hospital staff. Immediately after the birth the midwives gave the baby to them, wrapped but unwashed, supplied a tray of tea and left them to enjoy her for twenty minutes before returning to wash the mother and Sarah.

Those twenty minutes are remembered by the parents with happiness and gratitude. But when mother and baby were moved an hour later into the open ward, staff attitudes were different. As is not uncommon, the nursing was geared more to job efficiency and traditional practice than to facilitating what parents might want for themselves and their baby. Mothers were expected to conform to routines which conflicted with any wish for uninterrupted closeness, and most conformed.

But John and Jean had thought beforehand about the birth. They were agreed that the baby's place was with the mother, and were prepared to insist on this. Their view was reinforced by the unexpected strength of their protective feelings once Sarah was born.

So (though not without some trepidation in face of ward authority) they quietly but firmly insisted that the mother and not routine practice would decide when the baby would be in the bedside cot and when in the mother's arms. Sarah stayed close to her mother during the day, and throughout the night while other babies slept or cried in the night nursery.

It was difficult to maintain an attitude which conflicted with the orientation of the ward. Staff were not pleased; they kept up a steady pressure for conformity and were in minor ways obstructive. Jean held her ground, but the constant vigilance was tiring. Each new nurse had to be coped with afresh. Although of robust personality and not exhausted from a difficult birth she might have given way had her stay in the hospital been longer than forty-eight hours.

But the effort was worthwhile. When Jean came home with her baby, whom only she had handled in the hospital, she probably felt more at ease with Sarah than would a mother whose baby had been separated from her and fed and changed by nurses during the night.

When rigid attitudes interfere with a mother's natural feelings towards her new-born they add unnecessary tension and detract from the pleasure of a very special occasion. But as John and Jean have shown it is possible with forethought to overcome restrictions.

Fortunately there are maternity units which fully respect the wishes of parents.

Sometimes there is a medical reason for the baby to have intensive care. This will be distressing for the mother but of course the physical safety of the baby must take priority.

The parents, however, can if necessary make their concern about separation known to the doctors and nurses so that such handling or touching as is possible will help bridge the gap until the baby comes fully into the mother's care.

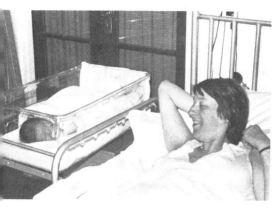

BABY SARAH is just $1\frac{1}{2}$ hours old, weight 9lbs. Jean is relaxed, and at first content just to look at her baby – amused by the great noise Sarah makes when sucking her fist.

After half an hour the mother took the baby into bed beside her, and when the baby began to nuzzle she put her to the breast. Sarah sucked for a minute and a half, then slept. Jean and John were delighted.

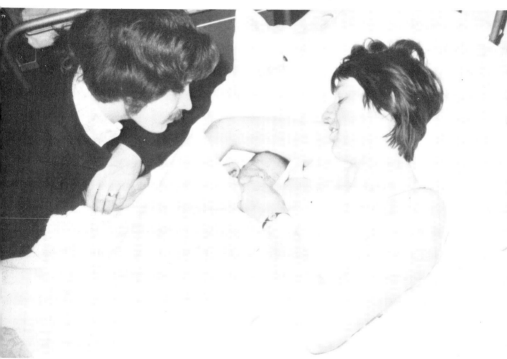

The nursing staff objected to the baby being put to the breast during visiting time in an open ward. They wanted the mother to wait for an hour to be 'instructed'. But the mother felt the baby was ready to go on the breast, so the father quietly drew the curtains around them.

As in most ordinary families a new baby holds everyone's attention – her every feature and movement seems miraculous.

The grandmother will stay in their home for two weeks to take over the domestic chores and so free the mother to attend to Sarah and get used to her new role.

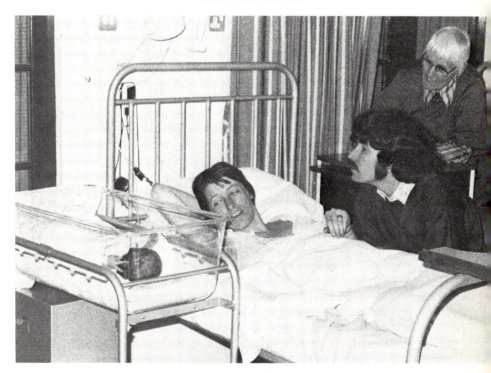

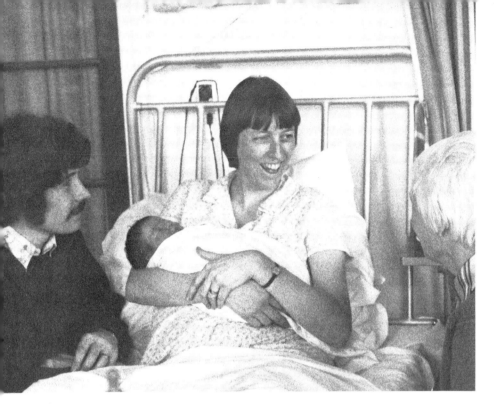

Sarah is 24 hours old. There is a cot at the bedside and a nursery next door, but the mother wants the baby near her night and day and for a great deal of the time in her arms. The closeness keeps mother and baby content. The parents have achieved what they wanted.

Unrestricted access to the baby reduces the tendency to tearfulness and low spirits which is common in new mothers.

Without the support of her husband she might not have been able to maintain her stand against the pressures of nursing staff for compliance with routine practice.

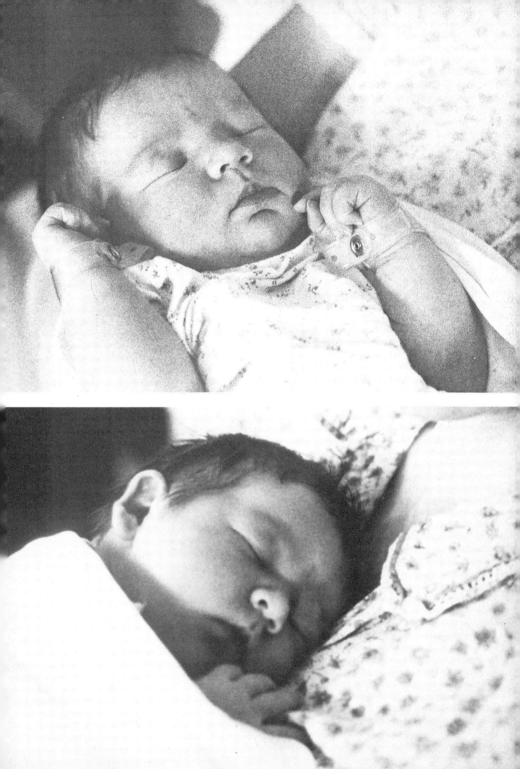

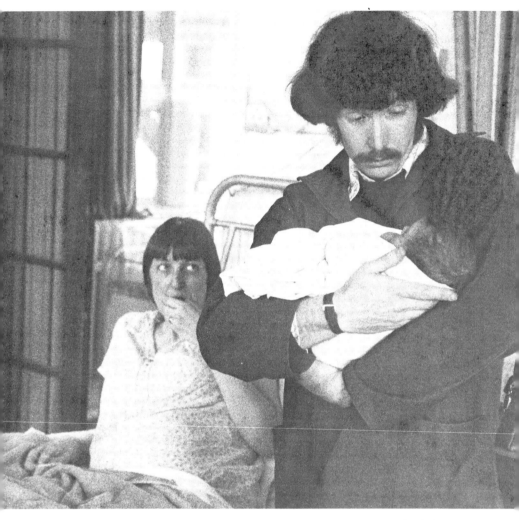

Father is unaccustomed to babies, and mother's eyes are on him with a mixture of pleasure and cat-like concern lest he drop the precious bundle.

Father feels joy, relief and anxiety in an uneasy mixture.

The First Few Weeks at Home

'One day I was pregnant – feeling special, being cared for and fussed over. Then suddenly I was home with a baby who had an insatiable appetite, who did not know that the night is for sleeping, and who dirtied all those nice new nappies.'

Jean

During pregnancy, parents-to-be dream about being together with a real live baby actually wearing and using all that lovingly prepared gear. In the elation of the run-up to the birth it is not easy to imagine the tiredness and lowering of spirits that can strike the mother afterwards.

In the early weeks, when the mother is at her lowest ebb, the baby needs a great deal of care. Just keeping him clean and fed takes hours and hours. No sooner is he settled after one feed and the mother has managed to have a snack herself than the next feed is almost due.

Feeding, whether breast or bottle, is a major preoccupation. Breast-feeding is most easily established by frequent small feeds whenever the baby wants to suckle. This is usually every one-and-a-half to two hours, with an occasional longer interval. The old idea of regular three- or four-hourly feeds is not suitable for a young breast-fed baby; to hold to such a routine means allowing the baby to become uncomfortable with hunger. It is much better to feed the baby 'on demand'; as he gets older and can take more milk the interval between feeds will become longer. Frequent feeding also stimulates the milk supply. **Bottle-fed babies must be fed according to a doctor's instructions.**

Whichever method of feeding is adopted it is a lengthy process which cannot be hurried. Sleep has to be snatched when the baby sleeps, and it is never enough!

Need for Help

Even when there are no complications in the birth, and no other young children to be looked after, the newly-delivered mother is often tired, anxious, and in need of support and assistance. It is wise to plan ahead for help in the home, and for ready access to someone who can sort out immediate anxieties about feeding, crying and sleeping which can throw the new mother into states of near panic.

Midwife, health visitor, grandmother, a friend with children, can fill the role. Family doctors expect to be called about new-borns. There are also self-help groups which have a telephone service that can give quick advice and reassurance which will calm anxiety. Very soon the mother's own feelings and experience with her own baby will be the best guide. She will learn from her mistakes and successes.

The most satisfactory help in the home is that which does not bring problems: a grandmother who deals with domestic chores and does not try to interfere with the mother's handling of the baby; a neighbour who does the shopping, but does not linger to talk too long; a home help who keeps out of the mother's way. If the father has paternity leave he will provide emotional support for the mother and an extra pair of hands to fetch and carry.

Anxiety and 'Baby Blues'

The high level of anxiety which is usual in the early weeks can be uncomfortable and frightening for the new mother, and confusing for the father because it is unexpected and not widely known to be common and normal. The mother may seem over-anxious about her baby, but the anxiety serves Nature's purpose by keeping the mother's attention focussed on the baby.

The anxiety may move into 'baby blues', or even into depression which needs medication, but usually it passes naturally within a few weeks.

'Baby blues' are much less likely if the mother has unhindered contact with her baby in hospital and in the early weeks at home.[2] An increasing number of maternity units recognize this and encourage the mother to stay close to her baby and handle him as much as she wishes. But some still do not, and the mother suffers pent-up frustration which can hinder her adaptation to the baby and may push her into low spirits.

To be relieved of domestic chores and protected from social demands during the first few weeks frees the mother to do what she most wants to do – to get to know her baby.

Difficulties Will Pass

Births do not always go smoothly. A prolonged labour or induction can leave the mother and baby sleepy and exhausted; after a forceps delivery mother and baby may be uncomfortable. Babies can be underweight or premature, or for some other medical reason need special care. There may be anxiety about a baby who is sick.

Help is then most important. The tiredness of an overburdened mother immediately affects the well-being of the baby. It is impossible to avoid all difficulties in the early weeks. Even when there are no complications there are adjustments to be made to the new family member and some tensions are inevitable.

But they pass, and what an achievement – a new life!

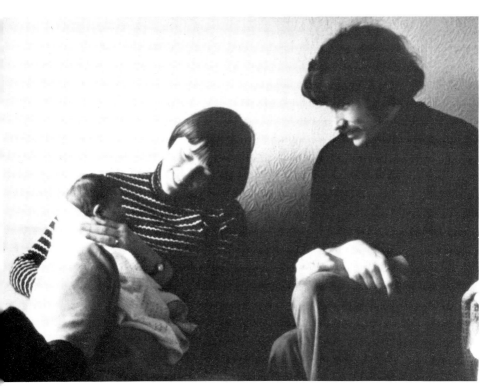

Home after two days. The long-awaited moment – now they are a family.

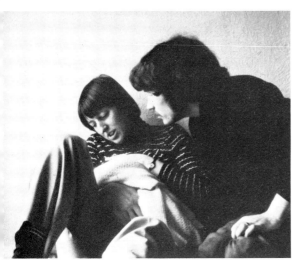

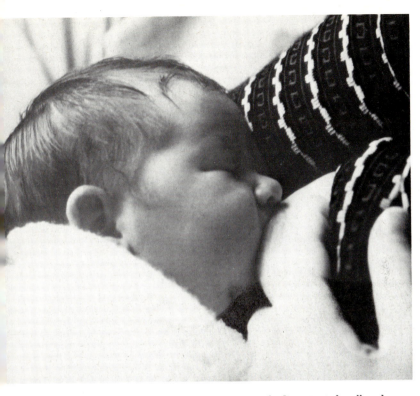

Breast-feeding started well and continued without problems. Sarah was put on the breast soon after birth and again whenever she showed signs of need; this was about every two hours. Sarah slept next to her mother's bed for six months, for as long as she needed night feeds.

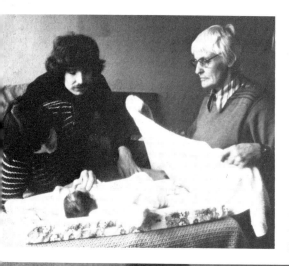

The parents can hardly take their eyes off Sarah. They marvel at her features, and at the well-shaped fingers that clasp theirs. There is a great deal of touching and looking.

The mother is pleased to have her own mother stay for a time, and welcomes practical help – especially with keeping nappies and shawls from falling off!

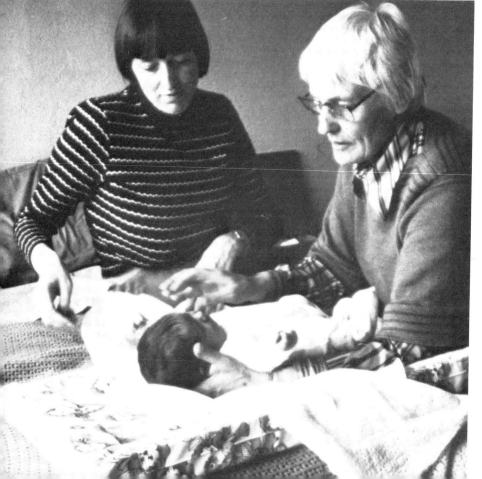

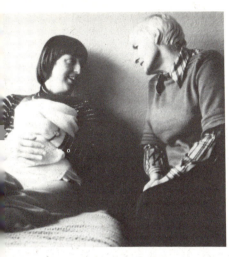

She is glad grandmother does not try to take over, but leaves her and the baby to find their own wavelength.

Mother needs to share not only her anxieties but also her pleasure in having a baby.

Grandmother cannot resist the pull of the baby and gets a turn at holding.

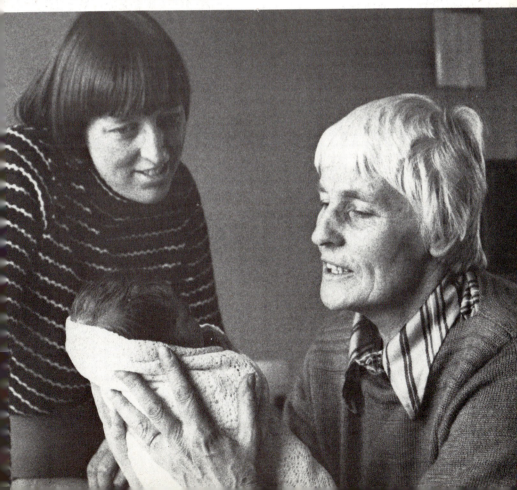

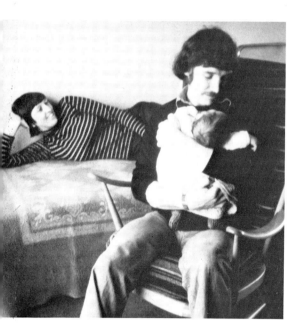

The father takes two weeks off work to help with domestic chores, but finds he wants to be useful in other ways! The mother is delighted that he is pleased with their baby daughter.

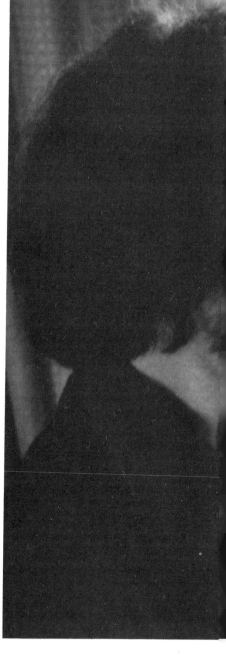

So-called 'baby blues' can often be eased by freeing the mother from domestic chores so that she can spend as much time as she wishes with the baby.

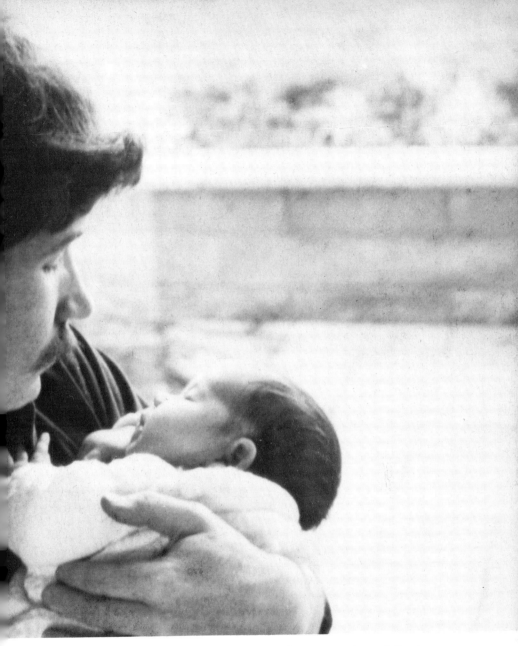

During his paternity leave, father is
drawn into the care of his baby.

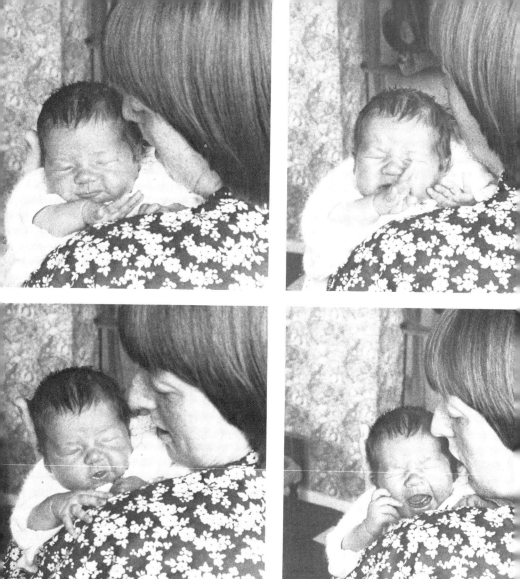

Sarah is 3 days old. It is not easy for
a young mother to understand and
meet the needs of a little baby who
screws up her face, looks very pink,
wriggles and cries.

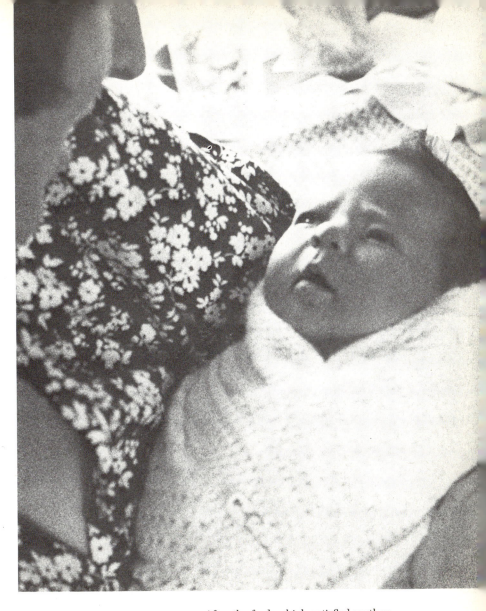

After the feed, which satisfied mother and baby, they gaze quietly at each other. This eye-to-eye gaze draws mother and baby together and is worth leaving the dishes for.

Parents can spend long periods watching, talking to, and touching their new-born baby; they are fascinated by the baby's eye-to-eye gaze, his smiling and movements.

But crying, which is as effective in catching their attention, calls out a different feeling – anxiety. A decision has to be made whether to pick him up or leave him to cry.

Sarah was never left to cry, because to her mother it seemed right and natural to pick her up and comfort her.

But some mothers are less sure of themselves. They may have husbands or parents or friends who warn against 'spoiling' the baby, or 'making a rod for your back'. Sometimes the fact that the baby stops crying when picked up is taken as proof that the baby was only pretending to be upset, or that he is pitting his will against that of the adult.

Crying is the only way a baby has to communicate distress. He cannot be 'spoiled' by being comforted. If his cries are answered he develops a feeling of trust in those who respond to him. (Even when there is no obvious need he enjoys being held close, to feel movement, or just to have company.)

Research has shown that babies who are left to cry tend to become grizzly one-year-olds, whereas those who are comforted are more contented. A comforted baby learns that his cries will be answered, but the uncomforted baby is uncertain that help will ever come.

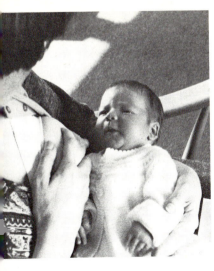

Just over 3 weeks old, Sarah is about to be fed. She breathes on the nipple or licks it, and waits for the milk to flow. Mother and baby are relaxed.

During the feed she looks up and smiles – as very young babies will do if they are full-term and closely mothered.

Play and 'talk' hold mother and baby together.

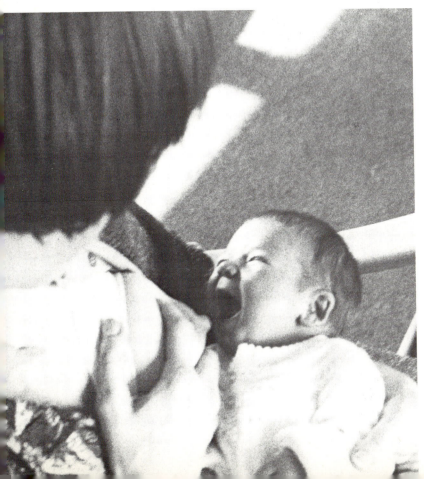

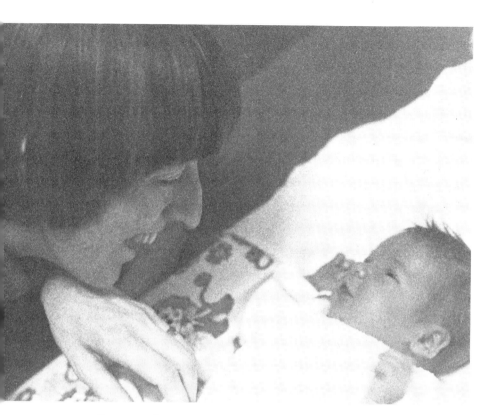

1 month

Mothers are impatient to get 'real' smiles of recognition.
The baby's smiles are irresistible – another aid to bonding. The sleepless nights and
mountains of washing fade into unimportance.

2 months

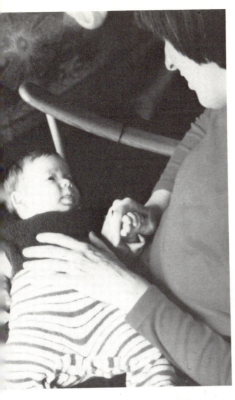

Mother thought the baby wanted a feed, but Sarah is content to 'talk'. The mother finds her gurgling as intriguing as her smiles.

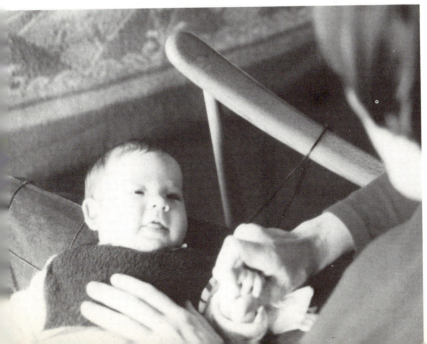

Then comes the feed.

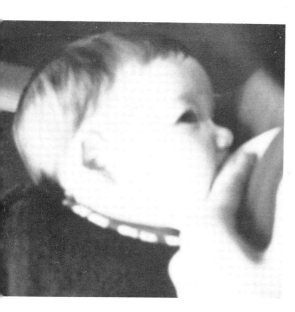

The feeding is over and Sarah is getting sleepy. Sucking her fist, she still looks at the mother's eyes and 'chats' to her.

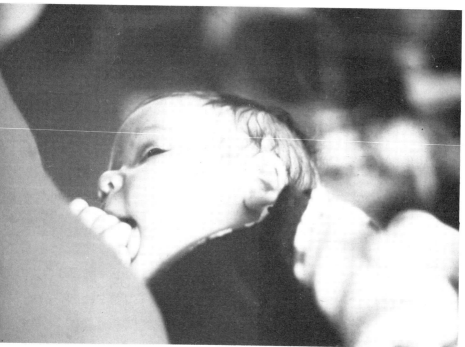

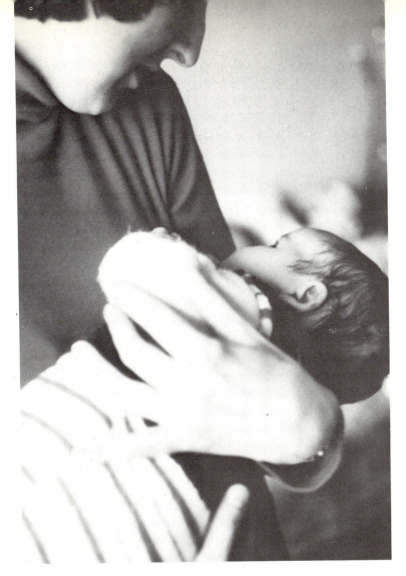

2 months

A baby can only look at the mother if the mother looks at the baby. If the mother turns away, the baby loses interest and turns away too.
A mother who is unable to give her baby time to gaze and gurgle misses experiences which deepen bonding.

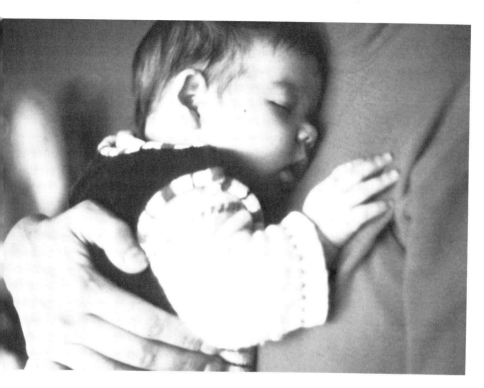

Although Sarah does not yet reliably recognize faces she knows the mother by her familiar handling, her voice, her smell. This gives Sarah a sense of security.

When the mother had 'flu she continued to breast-feed, but grandmother had to look after Sarah. On the second day Sarah became restless and calmed down only when returned to the familiar smell, touch and voice of the mother.

Continuity of care by the mother establishes in the baby a cluster of familiar sensations associated with her. This is an early stage of the baby's preference for the mother.

Chapter Two

The Love of a Baby for his Parents

(Sometimes called 'Attachment')

At around 6 months it is usual for a baby to cling to his mother, to cry if she goes out of sight or even if she moves too far across the room.

He is beginning to show clear 'attachment' behaviour. The presence of his mother has become necessary to his comfort and sense of security.

This is a gradual development which starts in less obvious ways in the early months.

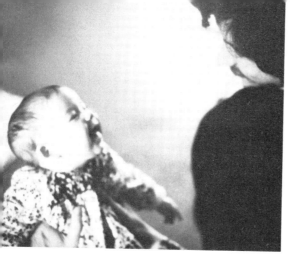

At 10 weeks Sarah smiles freely at her father and grandmother, making them feel ten feet tall!

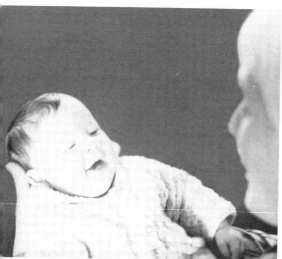

Lucy, the rag doll, also gets smiles and gurgles.

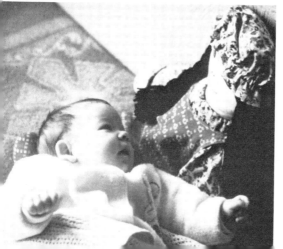

Any face with two eyes, a nose and a mouth attracts a baby of this age.

But for the mother Sarah also has a
grumbly cry which asks for
something only the mother can give
– the breast.

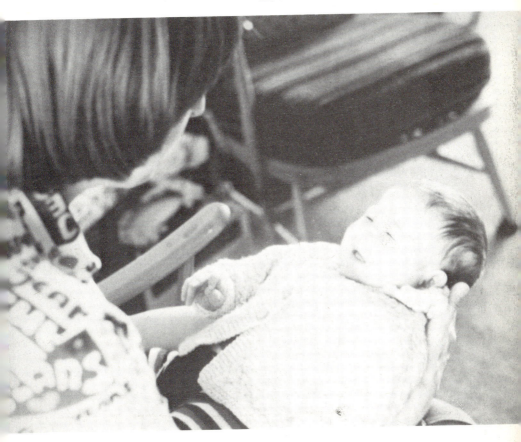

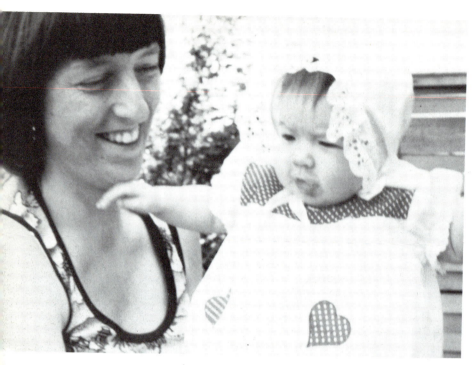

3 months

A typical 3-month-old, Sarah has a ready smile for everyone, and doesn't mind when people other than the mother hold her. She is everybody's friend.

But she is on the verge of a change.

$3\frac{1}{2}$ months

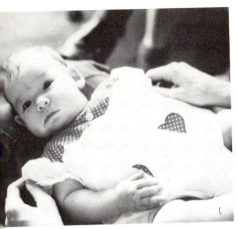

Just two weeks later Sarah begins to look seriously and searchingly at everyone including her father and grandmother.

She now sees the mother's face as different from all others.

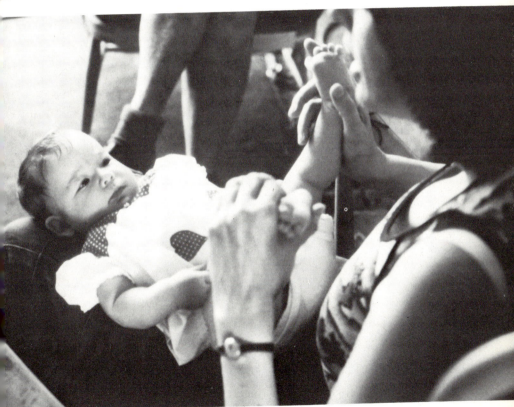

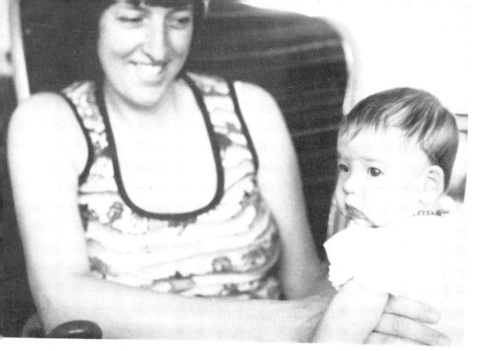

$3\frac{1}{2}$ months

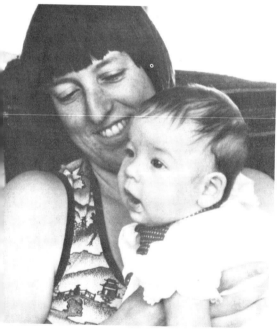

Although the grandmother has spent
two days each week with her since
birth, it now takes a few minutes
for Sarah to go to her.

Then she remembers where her mother is.

She is beginning to show a clear preference for her mother. This will grow stronger in the next few months and show vividly at about 6 months.

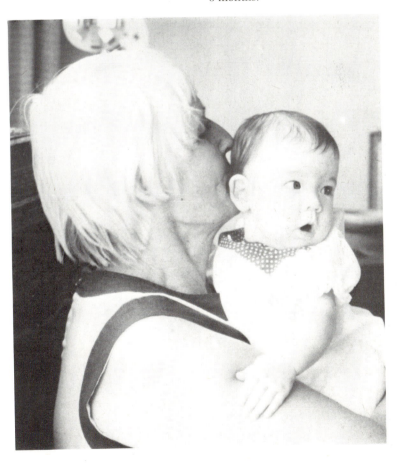

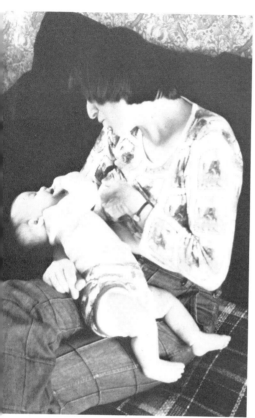
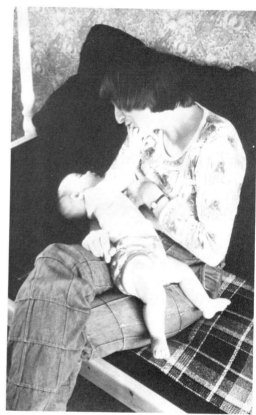

The mother enjoys answering
her baby's cues for food, for play,
for comfort.

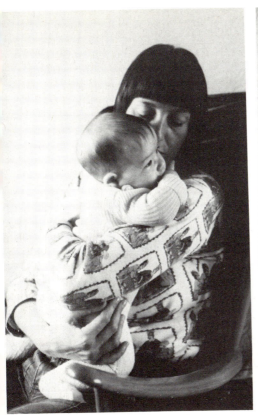
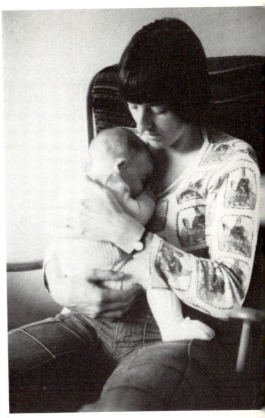

The sequence of being fed, playing at
the breast, and falling asleep is
repeated several times a day. This
repetition of good experience instils
in the baby a sense of security and
trust in the person who tends her.

5 months

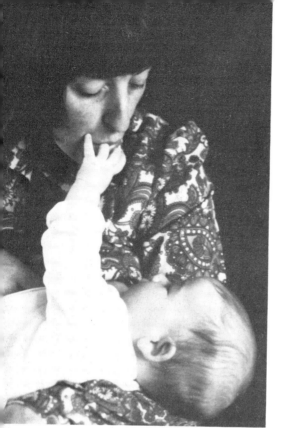

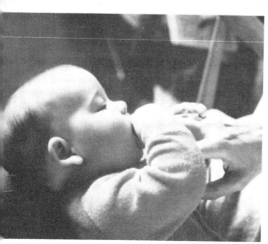

The mother is Sarah's whole life, and Sarah is a large part of the mother's life.

The relationship between them is close. The mother is 'in love' with her baby.

Each treats the body of the other as if it were her own. There are no boundaries between them. They 'eat' each other.

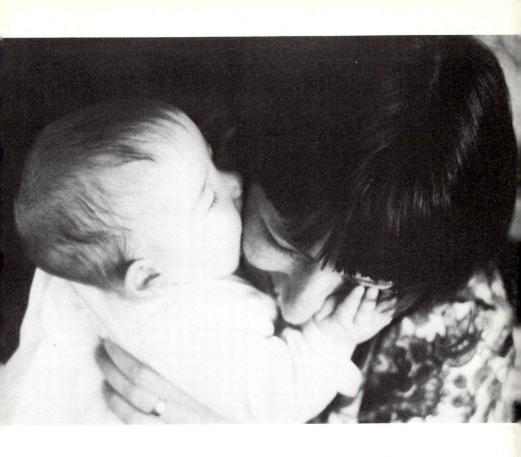

Some mothers resist early closeness to their babies, because they fear they will never escape from them. The opposite is true.

Such closeness in infancy is natural and essential. It gives the baby a secure base from which he can develop and gradually gain independence.

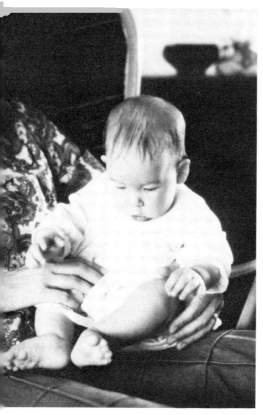

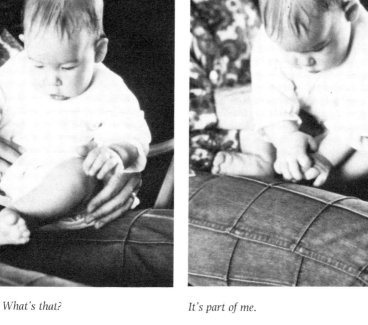

What's that?

It's part of me.

Sarah does not yet know that she is a
separate person. Gradually she finds
where her body begins and ends.

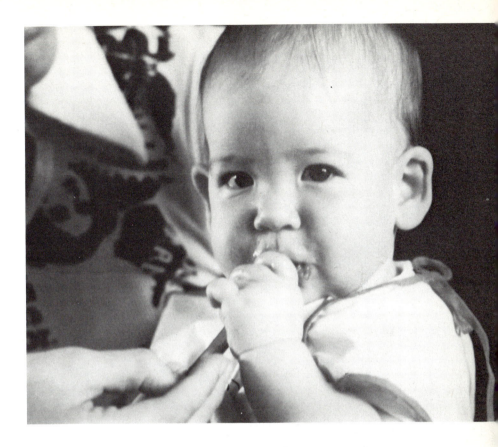

6 months

Crawling and weaning on to solid food are further moves towards separateness from the mother.

6 months

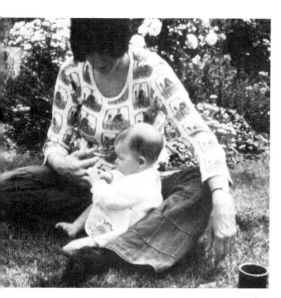

Mother helps Sarah find out more about the world beyond them both. Sarah wants to stand, but she cannot do it alone.

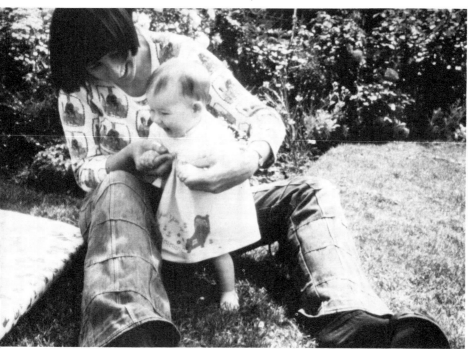

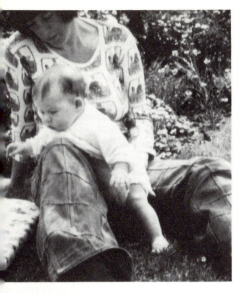

She tries to reach something and
again the mother gives just enough
help to enable the baby to get where
she wants to go. The mother lends
her hands, her arms, her knees, for
as long as Sarah needs them.

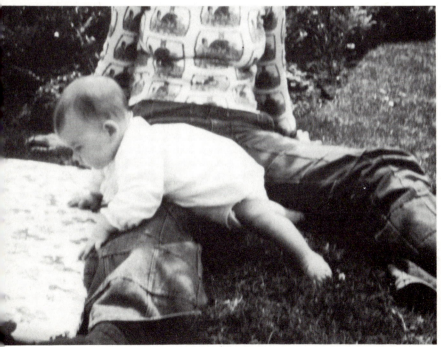

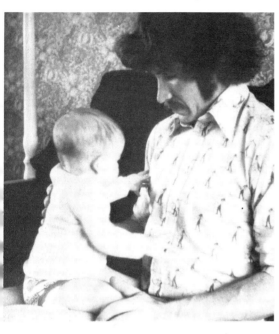

Sarah's relationship to the father is coming along the same paths as to her mother, but more slowly because she does not see as much of him.

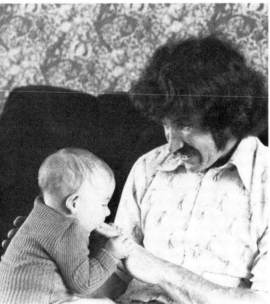

He gives her time to investigate him, to touch him, to mouth him as she does her mother.

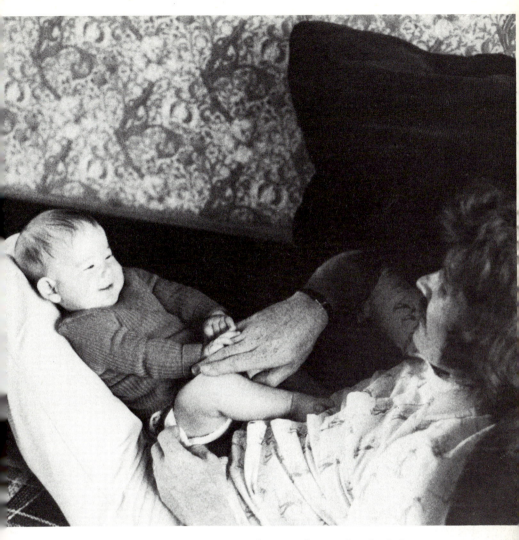

Father gets pleasure from his baby
daughter. He talks to her, listens to
and plays with her. He is protective
and 'in love' with her.

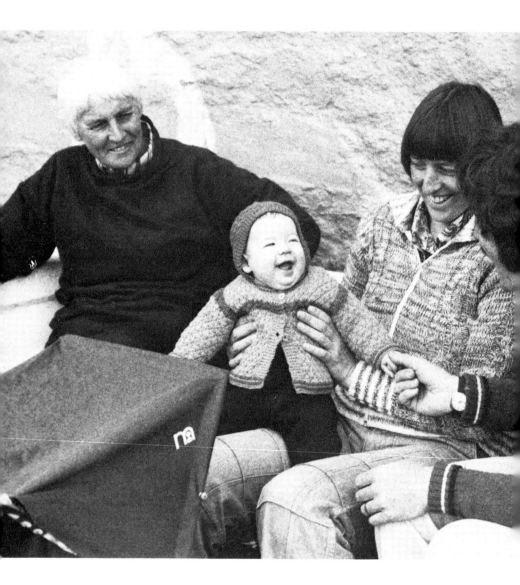

Sarah saw her father mornings, evenings, and at weekends. She did not know him as well as she did the mother who was with her all the time.

Sarah's relationship to her grandmother, who visited once a week and stayed overnight, was about the same as to her father.

But when the family went on holiday the extra time father and Sarah spent

$4\frac{1}{2}$ months

The family went on holiday for a week. The increased contact between father and Sarah added a richness to her growing attachment to him.

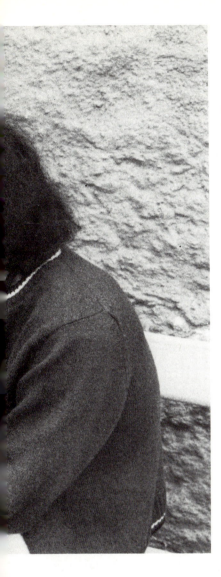

together increased her interest in him. Grandmother was relegated to third place.

The amount of contact between an adult and a baby is reflected in the baby's attitude to that person.

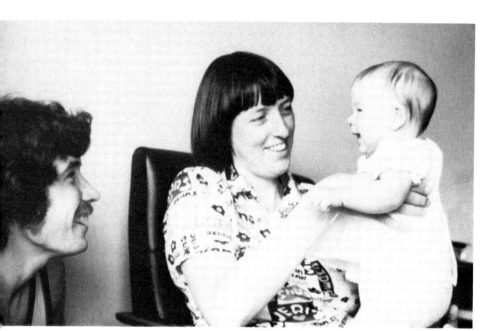

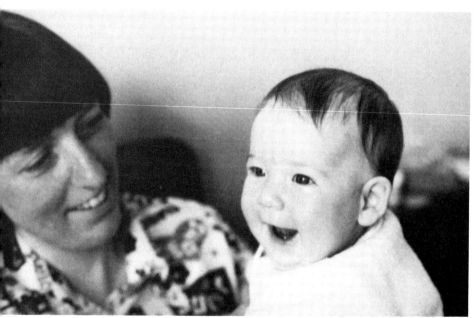

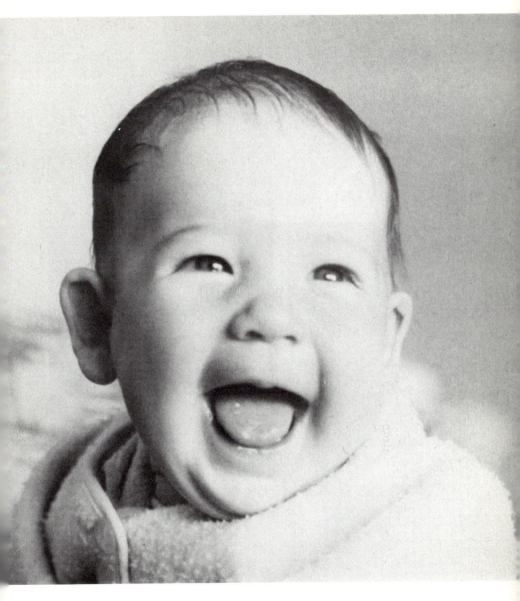

At home she saw her father for an hour or two each day, but on holiday she has him for most of the time. She greets him with the intense pleasure that is now reserved for her parents.

5 months

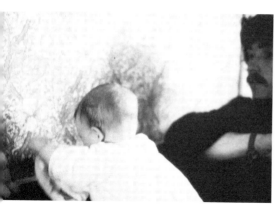

When they got home again, Sarah kept the warmth gained during their time together on holiday.

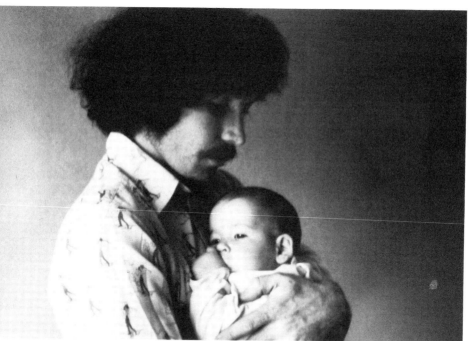

The father can comfort her, which she would not have accepted before the holiday.

This strengthens the bonding of father to her and Sarah's attachment to him.

Fear of Strangers

At around 6 months a baby loses his general friendliness and becomes wary, even frightened, of people outside the immediate family.

This lasts for a few weeks. Then the baby becomes friendly again, but only to people he knows.

It is an important step towards being able to make deep relationships with a few people and being reserved towards people who are not known.

Fear of Strangers

The period between 3 and 6 months is usually an easy time for baby and parents. Feeding has settled down and the baby may be sleeping for longer at night. He does not move far and can safely be left on the floor for short periods. He is nice to have around when visiting or being visited, because he is sociable and smiles at whoever stops to chat to him.

No Longer Everybody's Friend

But at around 6 months this delightful friendliness gives way to anxious tearfulness, and parents wonder what has gone wrong. '*Is he teething? Is he sickening for something? Or has he been "spoilt"?*'

It is none of these – the baby is growing up! He knows his parents and enjoys their familiarity. He has built around them and their ways of handling and talking to him a small world in which he feels safe. But now he is becoming aware of the world outside the family and he does not know how to cope with it.

At this time the baby's relationship to his mother becomes more intense, and he may cling to her. He is unwilling to be handled by anyone else, and fearful of people outside the family. He is no longer sociable, and cries if people overstep some safety distance which he alone knows. To touch him may cause panic. This phase of development is known as 'stranger recognition'. The baby now recognizes the difference between mother and other people, and feels safe only when close to her.

For the mother this can be a trying time, because the baby will not willingly be left with anyone – sometimes not even with the father.

Making Real Relationships

The fear of strangers usually lasts from two to six weeks, and varies in intensity from baby to baby. It gradually changes to a less anxious way of reacting to people he meets, then to degrees of friendliness according to their place in his life. He is more affectionate towards close family. To people outside the family, including relatives he sees infrequently, he is not immediately friendly; it takes time before he smiles or plays with them. There is a tendency to keep a distance from them, and to resist being touched or held. This often gives way to flirtatious behaviour, smiling from a distance then withdrawing if the person comes too close.

The baby is now beginning to show the social behaviour which will be expected of him later – strong feelings for his closest family, a lesser degree of friendliness to a few selected people, and a token social response to acquaintances. So 'stranger recognition' behaviour is an important stage of development. It is a step towards learning to discriminate between people, not a step backwards as is sometimes thought.

At the other extreme of care, a baby who spends much of the day in a crèche or day nursery where he is looked after by changing caretakers, and is not sufficiently with the mother to consider her special and different from all others, usually misses out this phase of development.

The result is a 7-month-old baby who does not cry at strangers, who remains friendly to all and accepts care from anyone, and who may seem the better developed baby. He is certainly easier to handle than a baby cared for by the mother. But the quality of his future relationships may undesirably resemble the quality of his present ones – shallow and undiscriminating. Such poor quality of relating if carried into adult life makes an unsatisfactory friend, colleague, spouse and parent.[3]

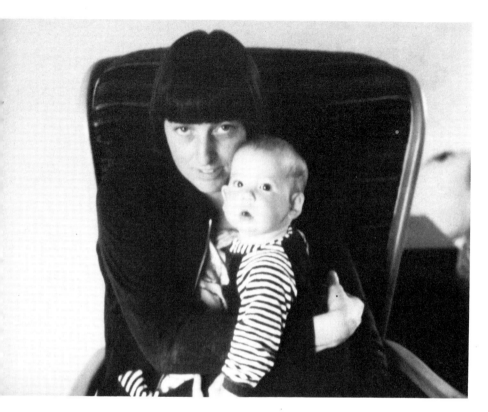

6 months

At about 6 months Sarah begins to cling to the mother and be fearful if anyone else comes near.

She has become aware of the bigger world beyond herself and her mother, and cannot cope with it. The only safe place is close to her mother.

These few weeks are difficult as Sarah goes through this phase. The mother understands Sarah's fearfulness and is prepared to shield her for as long as necessary.

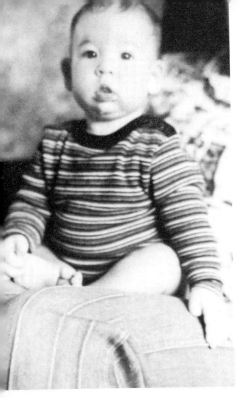

A month later the mother wonders if she has raised Sarah wrongly. It had seemed right to stay close to her, and Sarah had thrived on the closeness. But now the mother wonders whether Sarah will ever be friendly again, and father is a little hurt that Sarah has withdrawn from him.

Even Lucy, the doll, is viewed with anxiety!

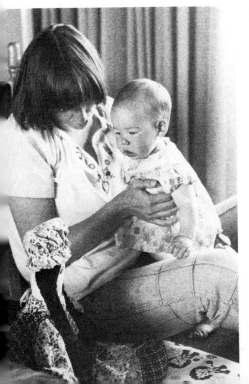

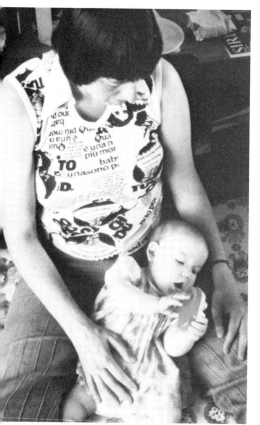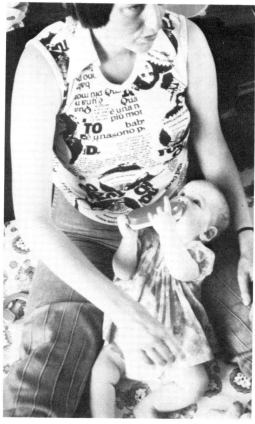

$7\frac{1}{2}$ months

The phase is passing. A visitor comes
to the home and, from the safety of
her mother's arms, Sarah can
tolerate the stranger's presence.
But had the mother moved away,
Sarah would have become upset.

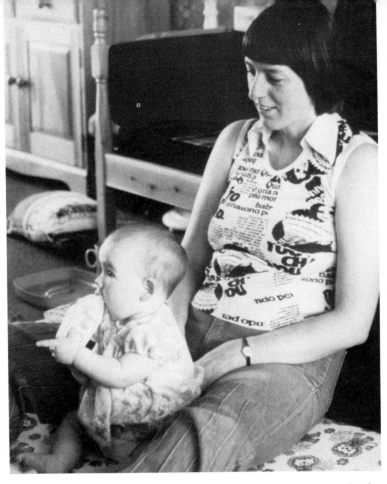

This has been a tedious time for the whole family.

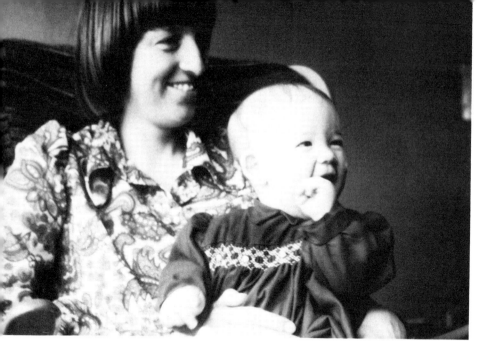

8 months

KNOWING THE FAMILY

At 8 months Sarah is friendly again to her father.

The family is once more relaxed and confident.

When he comes home in the evening she is excited to see him, and she loves to spend time with him in the mornings and at the weekend.

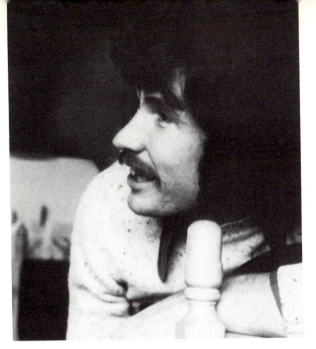

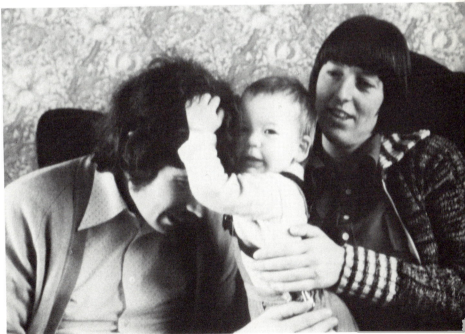

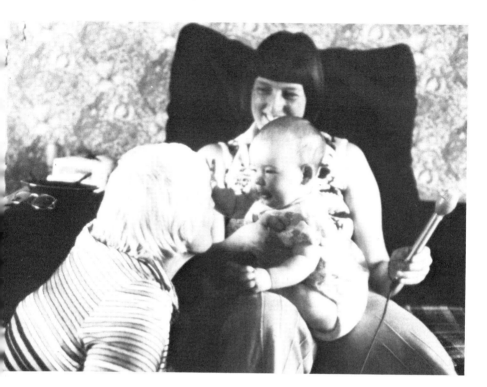

$8\frac{1}{2}$ months

Sarah, now $8\frac{1}{2}$ months, again
responds with pleasure to her
grandmother – but takes time to
touch and 'talk' to her.

After a short time grandmother is
acceptable. Sarah is then warm and
free of anxiety. They have fun
together.

Now that Sarah is again responding
to the family with affection, the
mother is more sure than ever that
she had been right to trust to her
own feelings in answering Sarah's
need for closeness.

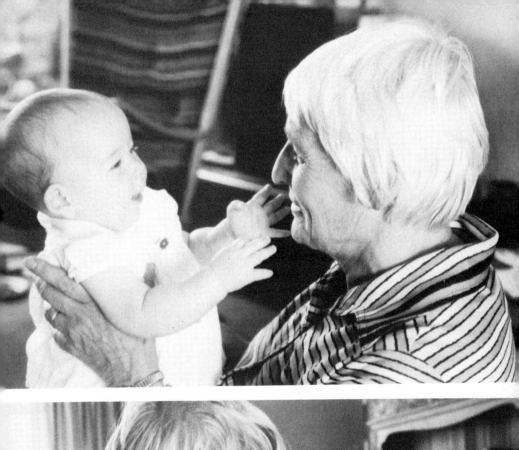
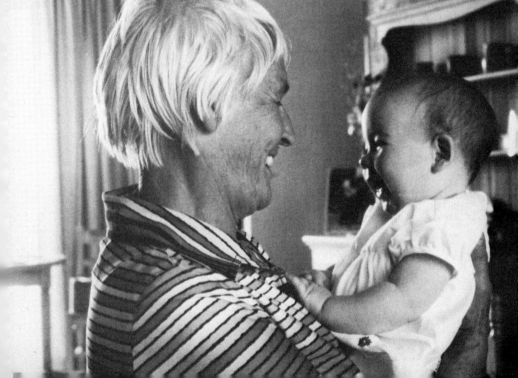

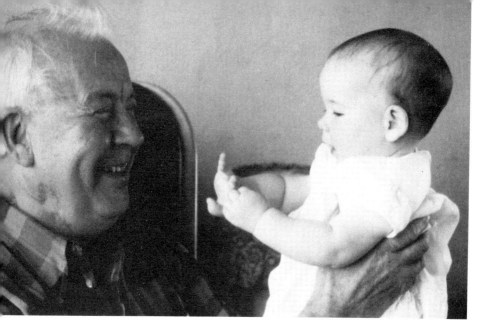

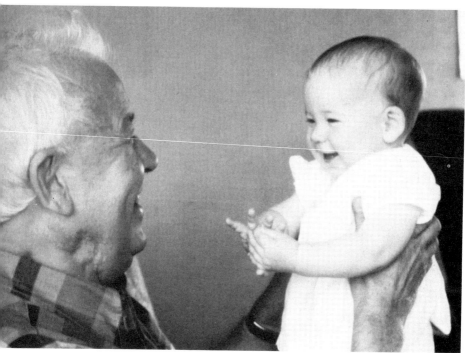

$8\frac{1}{2}$ months

The fourth person in Sarah's life is her maternal grandfather whom she sees once a week. She knows him less well and is slightly shy.

Within a few minutes she warms to him ...

... but when mother comes near, Sarah takes the chance to get back to her.

Visiting friends, especially those with children, are well tolerated; but they do not share the affection she shows to the family.

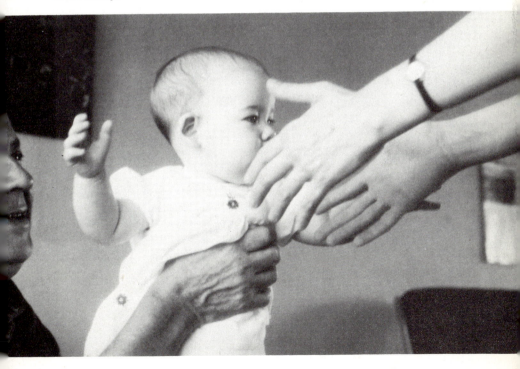

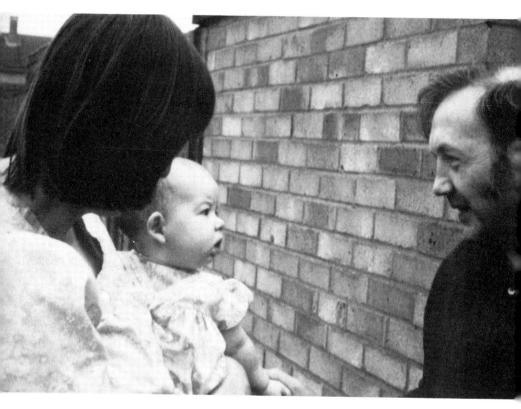

9 months

Sarah's other grandparents live at a
distance, so she treats them as she
would strangers. Her brow puckers
and she has no ready smile.

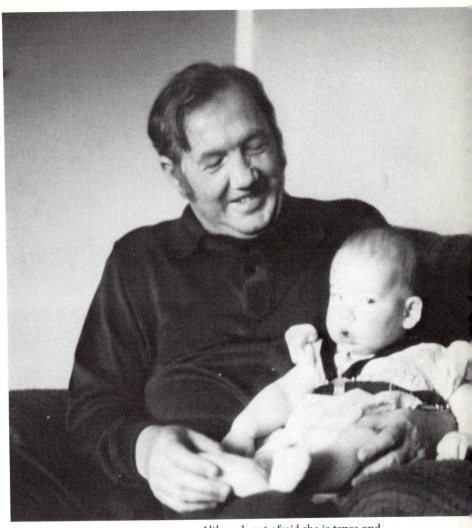

Although not afraid she is tense and uncomfortable. She doesn't want to be held by the grandfather she doesn't know – quite different from the friendly way she behaved on a visit three months earlier, before she began to distinguish between people she knew and strangers.

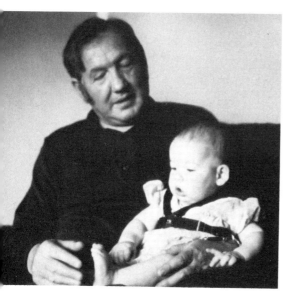

She doesn't want to be touched ...

... and pulls her foot away.

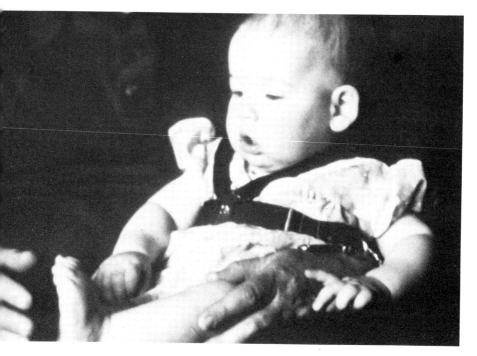

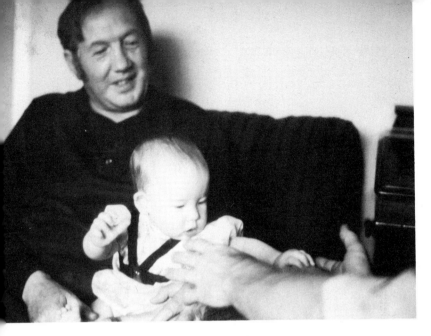

She escapes into her father's arms.

This behaviour in a 9-month-old baby towards her grandfather may be amusing, but Sarah is now distinguishing between people she trusts and people she doesn't know. When she is older it will be appropriate to have initial reserve towards strangers.

9 months

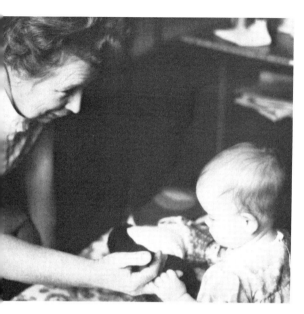

The paternal grandmother approaches slowly. She talks quietly and lets Sarah hold her hand before lifting her.

But Sarah needs more time to transform this unfamiliar grandmother from stranger into friend. There is tension in her face and fingers.

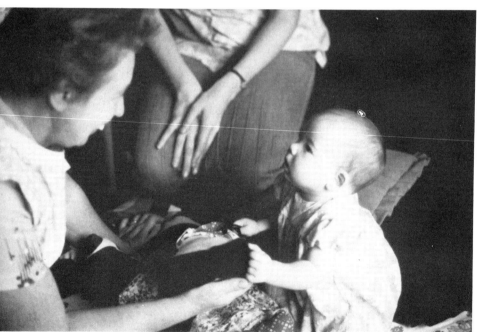

Sarah is uneasy and wants to get back to her mother. But by the end of the day she was at ease and friendly.

The grandparents who are seen infrequently will remain strangers until some time after Sarah's first birthday when she has the maturity to remember them from one visit to the next.

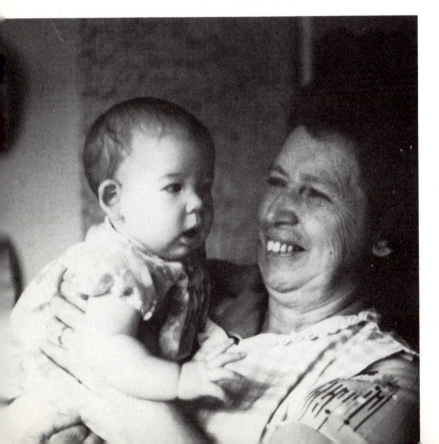

SETBACK
TO A RELATIONSHIP

Father injured his back and was in hospital for three weeks. In order that he should not disappear from Sarah's life, the parents 'bent' the rules so that mother and Sarah spent much of each day in the orthopaedic ward. But the father, being immobilized, could not respond to Sarah in familiar ways. For several weeks after returning home he still could not pick Sarah up and play with her as he used to. She reacted by becoming distant, treating him with cool friendliness. It was some months before the warmth and intimacy of their relationship was fully restored.

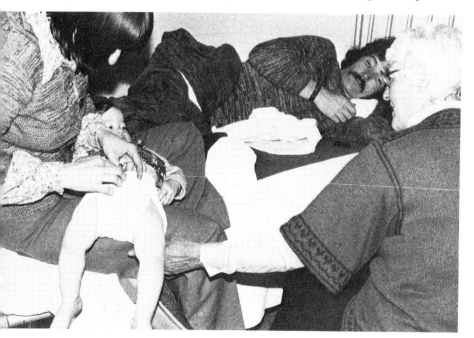

It is not only physical separation that a baby reacts to, but any withdrawal of affectionate interest such as may happen when a parent is preoccupied with illness, work, or worry.

Coming up to Twelve Months

Our account of the first year has concentrated on the emotional life of the baby and the quality of relationships.

But we now refer briefly to Sarah's attainment of skills, her feeding and her sleeping.

Milestones

At 1 year Sarah's functioning was excellent. She moved independently, crawling and walking round the furniture. Her noisy babbling had become a few recognizable words. She could make her needs known, and clearly indicate what she wanted – or equally important what she did *not* want.

Feeding

There was an allergic tendency on both sides of the family, so the mother was advised that for 6 months Sarah should be given *absolutely nothing – not a lick of anything – but breast milk* in order that the gut should mature, making an allergy less likely.

Sarah was therefore fully breast-fed for 6 months after which she accepted solid food with pleasure. She was weaned by 10 months and by 1 year was finger-feeding herself with a little help.

(At $2\frac{1}{2}$ years Sarah eats anything and has shown no sign of allergy.)

Sarah sucked her fist at birth then 'found' her thumb by about 3 months.

Sleeping

Like most babies she awoke two or three times in the night and needed a drink or a cuddle. So that everyone got as much sleep as possible, Sarah spent several hours a night in her parents' bed. She was never left to cry alone. She slept a 12-hour night (with breaks) and had a short sleep during the day. (The sleep pattern of a baby is rarely compatible with that of the parents. This is normal to early childhood, and there is no 'cure' other than for the baby to grow up.)

11½ months

Slow weaning from the breast was completed at 10 months.

Sarah 'helps' at mealtimes and enjoys finger foods.

She goes to the fridge when hungry, and indicates clearly when she has had enough to eat.

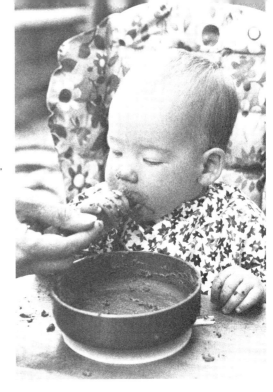

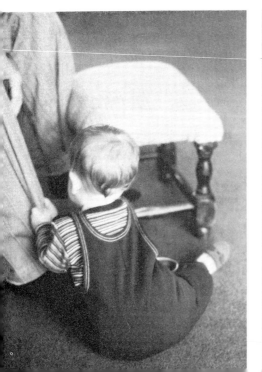

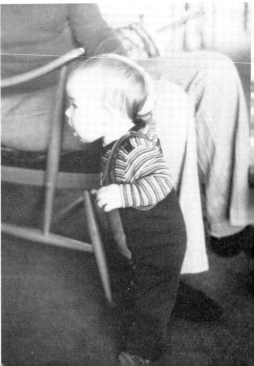

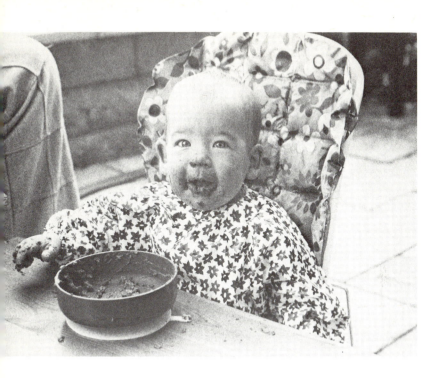

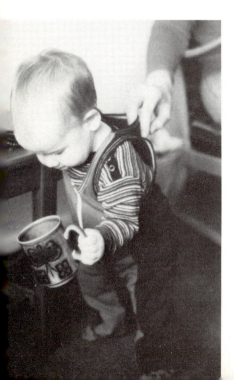

12 months
PURPOSEFUL PLAY

She uses her mother's trousers, then
the chair, to get to the coffee cup.

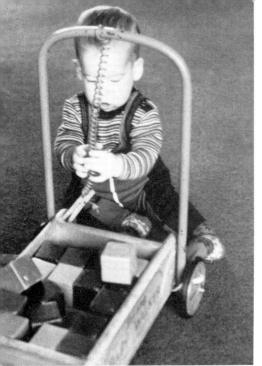

She concentrates on play.

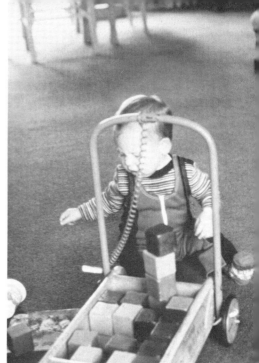

Something goes wrong and she calls for help.

CLARITY OF COMMUNICATION

At 12 months Sarah can communicate. She knows where to turn for help, and is confident of getting what she needs.

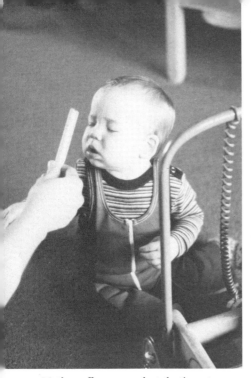

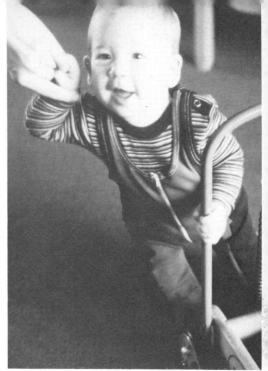

Mother offers a peg, but that's not what Sarah wants – so she goes on grumbling.

She wants to get up.

Now she can continue with play!

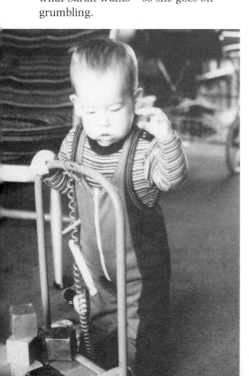

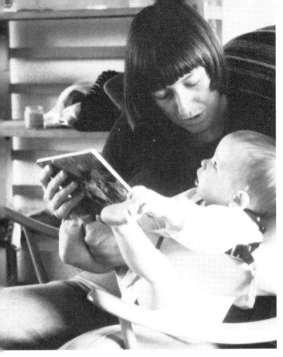

12 months

PLEASURE
AND CONCENTRATION

Sarah shows delight in her own body as
she curls up to share with her mother the
pleasures of a picture book.

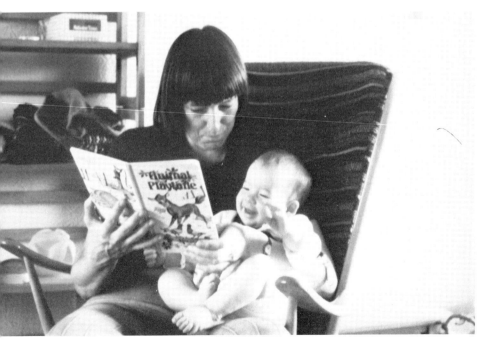

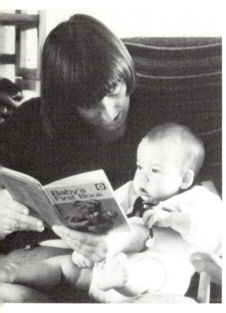

She listens and concentrates, and joins in with the animal noises her mother is making.

'-*ooff*!' for the dog is a favourite word.

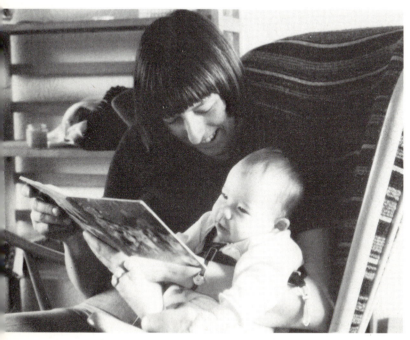

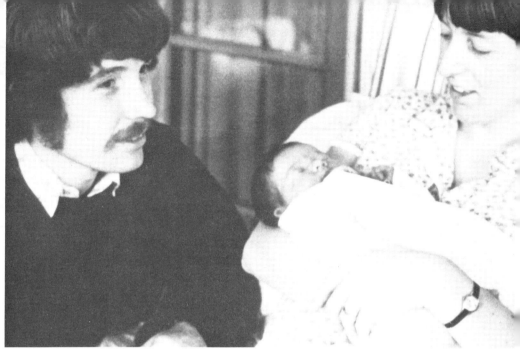

At the end of a year

Jean and John have moved from the
novelty of having a new-born baby
to a time when they cannot imagine
life without her.

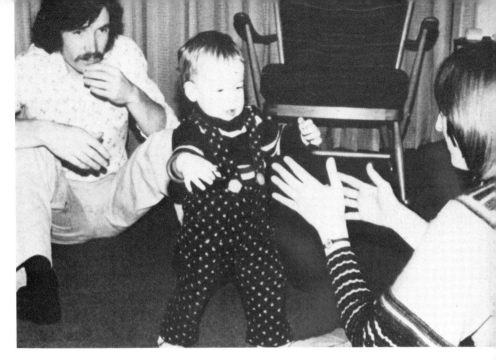

Throughout the first year Sarah's need for comfort, security and play had been met. At twelve months her serenity, her self-awareness, her curiosity and pleasure in the world around her, her ability to communicate feelings, reflect this early good experience.

The foundations have been laid, but like all one-year-olds she is vulnerable and her further good development depends mainly upon the continuing protective and facilitating environment provided by her parents.

Although Sarah appears robust, and within the family functions well, she is only a being in the making. She is a cluster of immaturities, and without the love of her parents she would soon crumble.

She has meagre language and comprehension, and a short memory; she cannot reason, cannot wait, cannot anticipate, and her feelings for people are not yet stable.

By about three she will be sufficiently independent to toilet and feed herself, and to make her needs known to someone outside the family. She will have enough sense of time to understand and tolerate a few hours' absence from her mother. She will then be ready for playschool, able to form a working relationship with teacher and other children.

Her ability to cope by herself with a bit of the world will have been achieved at her own pace and not thrust upon her prematurely for the convenience of adults.

Chapter Three

A Mother's Thoughts on the First Year

I enjoyed being married and childless. John and I sailed a boat, visited friends at weekends, and had holidays abroad.

I was a teacher and was very involved with my job. I spent hours planning trips out of school for the children. It was hard to imagine myself at home with a baby, so we delayed having a child for several years. The decision made, I was pregnant immediately. As the pregnancy advanced I became relaxed and less active in a way I could not have predicted.

All through my pregnancy I had one thing in mind – the birth. For months I was very apprehensive, but by reading and talking to friends and a gradual awareness of a real baby on the way I became more and more at ease. By the time labour was imminent I no longer worried – I took it all in my stride. In fact the baby was induced. Even that didn't bother me. I remembered all my relaxation and the birth was over at last.

But now I had a baby. I didn't seem to have thought much about that. The only things I was sure about were that I was going to breast-feed and I was going to keep my baby with me – even at night. As soon as the baby was born she was named Sarah.

I had read one or two booklets about babies. But all I seemed to have learned was that a baby should be fed at about four-hourly intervals, would probably cry with colic for some part of every day, and would very likely get nappy rash that needed a special cream from the doctor.

Now here I was with a baby, a real one that had not read the books that I had. Feeding was the first thing I had to have second thoughts about. Sarah was a natural at breast-feeding, and we had no problems at all. She was sucking her fist a few minutes after birth and at the breast two hours later. But she had ideas different from the books. She was not going to wait four hours between feeds. At first when I had no milk I let her suckle for practice. I had read that this was likely to help bring in the milk and give Sarah colostrum. But she also needed water because she was a big 9-lb hungry baby.

Night and day were the same to Sarah, and she wanted to suckle every $1\frac{1}{2}$ to 2 hours. The nurses did not object to this régime until it came to the night when I made known that I wanted Sarah beside my bed and not in the night nursery.

Sarah decided she wanted a feed or a cuddle every two hours or so throughout that first night. The ward sister got cross with me because I was getting so little sleep, and also because I had fallen asleep sitting up in bed holding Sarah. She suggested putting the baby in the night nursery.

I was tired, but by this time I had heard the heart-rending cries of other new-born babies in the nursery which happened to be behind my bed. Someone looked in on them frequently and fed them. But there was a lot of crying.

Sarah had given some short cries, but I had soon comforted her with a cuddle or a feed. I could not bear to think of her being left to cry for even five minutes when I could comfort her so easily.

The ward sister gave up trying to persuade me to part with Sarah and I was left to my own devices. Staff even abandoned trying to keep an accurate record of Sarah's feeds. I have no idea what they wrote down. I even began to lose track of feeds myself. But my Sarah wasn't crying, and that to me was important.

I was only in hospital for forty-eight hours, and when I went home I was lucky enough to have both John and my mother to help. I say 'lucky' because both were easy-going and prepared to do anything from changing nappies to cooking meals. Neither of them made any demands on me. My mother never tried to tell me how to look after Sarah, despite her experience, but helped me to learn about her.

John took two weeks off work. This we thought would give me company and let him help in the house. We didn't realize how quickly he would want to help with the baby – how quickly he would get 'hooked'. Together we watched Sarah for hours on end, unable to believe that this beautiful healthy baby was ours. Usually able to ignore any but the loudest of alarms, he found himself on duty during the night too.

For the first ten days I did not wash a nappy; I didn't cook a meal or do any housework. All my time was devoted to getting to know Sarah. I listened and watched to try to find out what she needed. I didn't want to do anything else. I was always ready with a cuddle or a feed. This had the result that I was still feeding very frequently, but the house was peaceful. Of course I was getting very tired, but I was pleased with the way Sarah and I were getting on. I was relaxed and happy. I was not tearful or depressed as I know some mothers are.

However, after a couple of weeks I was beginning to wonder whether we would ever be on anything less than two-hourly feeds and whether I would ever get a reasonable night's sleep. But with the support that my mother gave (she stayed for two weeks, leaving us alone for the weekends – and then for two days each week for a while) I managed to continue my sleepless existence. John often had to cook a meal when he came home from work.

This may sound dreadful, but we were all happy because Sarah was such a contented baby. She wanted frequent feeds but repaid us by smiling at us and looking alertly around. She rarely cried, often getting only as far as making a crying face and the odd grunt that signalled that something was wrong before she was picked up and cuddled or fed.

It wasn't until she was 6 weeks old that I began to get much in the way of sleep. By then she was gradually changing to 3-hourly feeds and the nights became more bearable. Things kept improving until at about 11 weeks she was on $3\frac{1}{2}$-hourly feeds (usually) and had one gap of 6 or 7 hours in the late evening.

My belief throughout Sarah's short existence so far was that if she cried it was for a reason, even if I couldn't fathom what it was. If nothing else helped I always managed to calm her with a breast feed. I was also more able to pick up the signs that heralded a cry. I hadn't accepted crying as an inevitable part of Sarah.

One other thing I did not accept as necessary was 'nappy rash'. Books seemed to describe cures but not prevention. One day I saw a very small patch appear. The doctor happened to call and prescribed a cream. However, I decided to try to find out what caused the rash.

The first couple of times a patch appeared it went without my finding the cause. Then the break came. John and I were thinking back to the other times it had happened and a pattern started to emerge – sherry one time, wine at another. Sure enough, next time I drank sherry the rash appeared for two days. So I rationed myself. It was worth it.

Later, after we had had a rough night I mentioned Sarah's restlessness to the visiting midwife. She said it might be something in my diet. She asked if I had eaten tomatoes or cabbage. I had. So from then on, in order to get as much sleep as possible I tried to work out what might have caused a particularly bad night. Often it was orange juice, tomatoes, cabbage, rhubarb, sprouts, or pickle. I cut these out from my diet for a while and got more sleep. Then I started to reintroduce them slowly, perhaps only three sprouts or a quarter of a tomato. I stopped again if it still seemed to affect Sarah.

My diet was rather restricted, but we were all getting sleep. Sarah's comfort and our sleep were more precious than food at this time. We were all getting along very well, and John and I couldn't imagine life without Sarah. But sleep was a commodity we were to be short of for a very long time.

The next few weeks passed pleasantly. Sarah thrived and John and I enjoyed her enormously – though we had our quota of colds and temperatures and anxieties.

We found that a sick baby is a worry like no other. A high temperature at midnight on Saturday when your doctor is off duty is Hell! Another new and unpleasant experience was to be ill myself, to have 'flu and still have to breast-feed an infant when all I wanted to do was look after myself and sleep.

But we managed. I was totally absorbed in Sarah, and surprisingly did not wish for anything else.

Around 7 months, when Sarah was unwilling to be touched by anyone and clung to me day after day, I did feel fed up and unsure that I had been doing the right thing by allowing Sarah to be so close to me. Yet at the same time I couldn't think where I might have gone wrong.

I was reassured to learn that most babies go through this phase and that it would soon be over.

John was as interested as I was in every new development, and we discussed the problem of Sarah's clinging and any other that cropped up. It was a relief when she got over this patch and we could all relax again.

From then on Sarah began to show more independence in lots of ways – crawling, walking around the furniture, eating solid food – and I was breast-feeding much less. She did not need so much attention and I was getting impatient to follow some of my other interests.

I had to find ways of coping with my bouts of boredom.

I tried to make sure I went out every day – shopping, visiting friends, and to the park. I took up the simple craft of macramé because I could leave it at any point and Sarah could pull at the string and do no harm. Lace-making was out of the question.

We live on a small housing estate and our nearest relatives are sixty miles away. Towards the end of the first year I was getting desperate to meet people, but had to delay going to mother–toddler group until the summer when Sarah was 16 months; there was a whooping-cough scare and Sarah had not been vaccinated because of a possible allergic reaction.

The mother–toddler group, baby swimming group, and meeting friends with children has filled some of the gaps. But I am looking forward to the time when I can think my own thoughts without the constant chatter of toddlers.

Although my brain seems to be in cold storage, and my concentration not what it was, I am looking after Sarah in the way I want to. She gives us enormous pleasure and we are proud of the way she is developing.

JEAN

Chapter Four

Parents – Trust Your Feelings

Parental intuition to stay close to the baby is in accord with modern understanding of the needs of babies and families.

Some maternity units and paediatric wards provide for this. But some do not.

So it is important for parents to know what they want, and if necessary to take a stand. If the need arises, it is not that the parents are over-anxious but that the hospital's attitudes are out of date.

Paediatrics is concerned with something more than nursing and the treatment of children. It includes encouraging the mother to develop her own skills by which she remains the chief instrument of child care. The mother is equipped for her duties by developing sensitivities to danger beyond the range of normal feelings. She will hear the whimper of a child in a distant bedroom when other ears are deaf. She will awake instantly to the needs of her child when strangers would do no more than stir slowly in their sleep.[4]

Sir James Spence,
Nuffield Professor of Child Health

In the Maternity Unit

Most parents feel close to their babies, and are as protective as the parents of Paul and Sarah. They are sensitive to the absolute dependence of the baby, and seek to avoid the distress to both mother and baby that would occur if they were separated.

Hospital practice is slowly catching up with parental intuition and current knowledge of family relationships. Studies have confirmed the importance of early and continuous contact between mother and baby, and of the early involvement of both parents.[5] In a growing number of maternity units it is now clearly understood that routines should not unnecessarily intrude upon the wishes of parents to be close to their new-borns; and that, no matter how 'fussy' the behaviour of a mother may seem, this should not be obstructed except in the rare circumstance that it endangers the physical well-being of her baby. She and the baby have a long time ahead after they leave the hospital, and however idiosyncratic the relationship is going to be it will have its most positive beginning in a ward which helps the mother to get to know her baby in her own way.

The philosophy of the better maternity units is that the baby belongs to the parents and not to the staff. In some wards this is quite explicit with reassuring notices on the walls like this one: '*Babies and mothers know best about breast-feeding. Babies can be breast-fed whenever and for however long they want.*'

Parents who find themselves in such an enlightened ward will fit in easily and with none of the tension experienced by Jean and John.

But even in the most enlightened of maternity units there can be lapses – a new nurse who doesn't quite understand, a new registrar who doesn't fully share the consultant's views – so the parents may on occasion have to give a nudge to the system to ensure that it consistently meets their wishes.

Not all maternity units yet run in accord with present-day knowledge of the importance of parenting.* It is then of great advantage if before the birth

*A complaint by parents that a special-care baby unit had unreasonably restricted access to their baby was upheld by the Health Service Commissioner (Ombudsman). He drew attention to Health Service Circular HC(78) 28 of 1978 in which authorities are advised that babies who have to stay in hospital are particularly vulnerable to their families losing contact, and that 'wherever possible facilities should be provided for the mother to stay in hospital with the baby; failing that it is important that the parents of these babies be encouraged to visit and play a part in caring for them'. The Area Health Authority concerned were 'invited' to review their practice about access.[6]

the parents are clear about their wishes, so that whenever necessary they can confidently refuse to allow the persistence of outdated restrictions to come between them and their baby. As with John and Jean their forethought will be strengthened by the surge of protective feeling that arises when they hold the baby for whom they have waited so long.

A successful stand against unnecessary restrictions can be taken if it is remembered that the nurses are not ogres but ordinary mortals operating a system of care which has not yet caught up with the times. No one will evict parents who insist on the baby staying close to the mother.

But when, as happened to John and Jean, the nursing staff maintain a resistance against the parents' wishes it can undoubtedly be difficult for the mother to oppose hospital authority as represented by the uniformed ward sister.

The Sick Baby in Hospital

Although parents hope their baby will never have to go into hospital, and commonly close their minds to the possibility, it is wise to acknowledge that this could happen and to have a clear idea of what they would want to do.

The better paediatric wards respect the family unit and fully involve parents in the care of their sick baby. The mother is encouraged to stay in the same room as the baby, night and day, to meet his mothering needs and prevent the distress of separation from her while the staff concentrate on making him well again.

But not all paediatric wards have yet reached this level of family-centred care, so it is prudent of parents to take the precaution of discovering where the best hospital care for children is to be found in their region. There are organizations which can give this information.[7] Then if unfortunately the baby has to go into hospital they will know where to take him in confidence that their natural anxiety and wish to stay close will be understood and provided for.

But if they find themselves in a ward which is restrictive it is essential to remind themselves that this vulnerable little person to whom they have given love and responsive care belongs to them and not to the hospital. And that, as far as the medical condition allows, they wish to give him the comfort of their familiar presence and care. It is also important for the bonding of the mother in particular that she be there. They will not be put off by assurances that if they leave the baby he will 'settle'. Research has shown that the baby who is left alone in hospital may indeed go quiet and be easy for the nurses to handle, but his security will be shaken.[8]

But parents do not need research findings to tell them what is best for their baby. The thought of how the baby will feel if shut off from the comfort of the mother's care, especially when he is ill, will sweep aside the traditional assurances they are likely to be given in a restrictive ward. Their task is to hold firmly to what they want for their baby, and not to be moved from that by any suggestion that they are 'over-anxious'. If the ward does not have beds for them, most parents will be content to sit all night by the cotside rather than leave the baby alone. Better still, they will bring in their own folding beds or reclining chairs – confident that this is wholly justified by their proper concern for the baby's emotional well-being and that many other parents have done this before them.

But it is not easy to take a stand against hospital authority, even if it is only that of an unsympathetic ward sister. A mother who is anxious about her baby's illness may be in danger of being intimidated. Father is a necessary support for her and often the best person to talk to doctors and nurses.

Disagreeable though it may be to face staff displeasure in an outdated ward, parents will be doing no more than requiring facilities recommended by the Minister of Health.[9]

Parents who hold to what is best for their baby will by their example help soften attitudes to other parents.

The Sick Parent in Hospital

If the mother or father is a patient in hospital this is another instance where the baby's close relationships have to be safeguarded. Sarah spent time with her father when he was in hospital. John and Jean discovered that in the orthopaedic ward the staff were able to accept mother and baby as visitors for much of the day.

Sustaining contact is even more important if the mother is the patient. She is the one who is closest to the baby, and whose absence will affect the baby most.

Visiting may not be possible for some days, but as soon as the mother is well enough it is highly desirable for the baby to be with her as much as is practicable – certainly for much more than the limited visiting hours which usually apply in adult wards.

Full family-centred care will be the care of the future, and parents who make a stand now against unnecessary restrictions will help bring this about.

For such periods as the baby may not be with the mother in the hospital it is important that he be looked after by one person only who will handle him in ways as similar as possible to those of the mother, answering the baby's cues for attention, and being tolerant of any upset shown by the baby because of the separation.

The best caretaker is often the father, taking time off from work. Otherwise a close friend or relative or foster-mother who can devote herself full-time to the task – beginning, if possible, in the days before the mother goes to the hospital.

Chapter Five

What We Mean by Bonding and Attachment

There are two separate parts to the parent-child relationship.

'Bonding' refers to the feelings parents have for their children, and 'Attachment' to the feelings children have for their parents.

Although they run in parallel, bonding and attachment begin at different times, have different qualities, and different outcomes.

To see them in this way aids our understanding of family relationships.

Bonding: *The Feelings of Parents for Their Babies*

Parents feel their own children to be special and make allowances for their shortcomings, make special efforts for them, share their experiences, are sad for them, are happy with them. They even find their naughtiness has a curious appeal, and they reserve the sole right to be angry with them.

Parents' preference for their own children is quite irrational, having little to do with their actual qualities. This irrational love has to be experienced to be appreciated. When seen in others it can irritate. Before having their first baby a young couple can be puzzled by the behaviour of friends who have a child. These friends may have been level-headed and interesting to talk to, but after having a baby they seem to talk too much about their offspring and to plan their lives too much around him. They may appear over-anxious, over-protective, possessive, besotted, indulgent.

Not until the couple have a baby of their own can they understand the behaviour of their friends. They find themselves caught up in similar feelings which they could not have anticipated. They begin to be 'bonded'.

'Bonding' is increasingly recognized as a major force in keeping families intact, in safeguarding children from parental abuse and abandonment.

Mother and Baby

The bonding of mother to baby occurs most easily when conditions during and after the birth are right – when mother and baby are kept together, when the mother can see and touch the baby and answer to his needs, when there is the intimacy of breast-feeding, and when she has the love and support of her husband.

It is not only because she is the principal caretaker that the mother becomes deeply bonded. Within a day or two after giving birth, most mothers experience an upsurge of anxiety and tearfulness. The intensity varies from one woman to another. The anxiety springs mainly from hormonal changes triggered off by the birth; it serves Nature's purpose of safeguarding the baby by keeping the mother's attention focussed on him.

The mother is specially alert to the baby; she cannot ignore his cry, which she feels as much as she hears. Each time she answers the baby's need for attention, each time she comforts or feeds him, each time she holds him – has him look into her eyes, has him curl his fingers around hers – she feels more necessary to him. The baby's survival depends upon the mother's care, and this knowledge adds to her anxiety and to the tightening of the bond.

In the early days and weeks, the more opportunity she has of being the person who answers the baby's needs, who knows him better than anyone else, who is the one he depends upon more than any other, the quicker and stronger the bond will develop.

If breast-feeding is established this brings mother and baby closer still, partly because of the intimacy and partly because of the hours that are spent in feeding.[10]

If hospital provisions and family support have kept the mother–baby couple together, by the time the heightened anxiety lessens (at around eight weeks) the mother is unreservedly 'in love' with her baby.

The Appeal of the Baby

At first the baby's contribution to the bonding of the mother is his appealing helplessness, but he soon has other means of drawing her to him. By about the third or fourth week (often even earlier) he begins to smile, then to gurgle and coo. Few adults can resist a smiling, babbling baby – least of all she who has waited nine months to give birth to him.

As the bonding deepens the mother is more and more convinced that hers is indeed a very special baby. Her pleasure and pride in caring for and 'owning' him, in sharing and facilitating his development, compensates for the disturbed nights and the setting aside of her own wishes in favour of the baby's needs.

Need for Early Contact

The foregoing account presumes a mother who has had a good confinement, early access to her baby, and a ready response to him. But bonding also occurs when the mother has had a bad confinement, perhaps coupled with a delayed response, or when the baby is ill or handicapped, provided contact between mother and baby is begun without too much delay.

Bonding of the mother will be interfered with if the baby is left in hospital without her. The better special-care units recognize that delay in getting parents and baby together can be detrimental to the baby's development and to the quality of the parents' relationship to him. For this reason they encourage mothers to stay with their premature, sick, or small babies, and to feed and handle them. Mothers who cannot stay visit frequently.

Father

Many a modern young father is in close contact with his baby. He shares in the baby's care and becomes deeply bonded. But the father's bondedness is unlikely to be as compelling as the mother's, because much of his day is spent away from home and his involvement with the baby is therefore less.

It is just as well that fathers do not become quite as bonded as mothers, since fathers have to go to work. They must be able to resist the baby's cry, and later the toddler who pleads: *'Don't go to work. Stay home with me.'*

But when necessary, for instance if the mother is ill, the father who has helped in the care of his baby is usually the best substitute for her.

Grandparents

Grandparents become bonded to a degree reflecting the amount and quality of their involvement. But except when they are the child's caretakers (for example during a mother's prolonged illness or when a mother is in full-time work) the bondedness of grandparents will be much less than that of parents.

A degree of grandparent bonding is useful in providing a safety net for the young family.

Adoptive Parents

The baby who is adopted in the first few weeks of life will stimulate feelings in the adoptive mother comparable to those of a mother who has given birth. Although the special level of anxiety caused by hormonal changes will not occur, anxiety will nevertheless be aroused by the helplessness of the baby and by her responsibility for keeping him safe and well. The cries and gestures of the baby are genetically designed to elicit pangs of love and concern, and as she cares for him the adoptive mother will be carried into a high degree of bondedness.

This indicates the importance of direct placement into the care of the adoptive parents, and is an argument against the common practice of using the intermediate care of a foster-mother or residential nursery. Adoptive parents are already at some disadvantage because the baby has not been born to them. Every week of delay in making the placement is a loss of important early experience leading to satisfactory bonding.[11]

If the baby is taken over after the first year, bonding is likely to develop less strongly; and, because the adoptive mother has not been exposed to the irresistible appeal of the baby's behaviour in the first months, the bonding will lack something of the fullest commitment. In the year preceding placement for adoption the baby's ability to attach may have been impaired by multiple care in a residential nursery, or by the loss of a loved foster-mother.

Deferred placement for adoption is undesirable. With time and patience on the part of the adoptive parents, mutual affection between them and the baby can be built up; but the relationship is unlikely to be as deep and satisfactory as one developing from direct placement in the first few weeks of life.

Attachment: *The Baby's Feelings for His Parents*

a. Birth to about 6 months: Everybody's Friend

The new-born baby cannot at first make sense of the world. But as his mother handles him day after day in familiar ways a pattern begins to emerge. Each time she picks him up he recognizes her smell and touch and voice, and soon learns that feeding or comforting follows.

Within the small world she thus creates for him the baby 'knows' the mother in these primitive ways, and in time she becomes the person he can distinguish from the more fleeting people who come and go.

At about three months he recognizes her face clearly, where previously he sensed only her familiarity, and he responds to her with greater animation than to others. But throughout most of the first six months the baby is friendly and smiling to everyone, and allows himself to be held by almost anyone.

It is part of the parents' pleasure in their baby at this time that his friendliness draws appreciative comments from acquaintances. But, generally friendly though he is, the baby is gradually developing a specially intense response to his mother.

b. About 6 months: Fear of Strangers

At about 6 months his behaviour changes quite dramatically. He clings to his mother; he wants her and her alone, and cries when strangers approach him. She has become his haven of safety. Father and grandparents may find themselves shunned and avoided. Father can feel a pang of hurt that his baby is unwilling to stay with him, and the grandparents may be puzzled and even impatient that the cherub will no longer sit beaming on their knees. The baby dislikes being apart from the mother, and cries if left in a pram outside a shop.

This is not a step backwards and the baby has not been 'spoilt'. The recognition of strangers is an important step in the baby's development.

During the previous months his mother had shared his pleasures and anxieties, tended him during illness, aided him in the gradual mastery of his body, understood his non-verbal communications. This and their physical closeness has established her as the most familiar person in his life, the person he enjoys most being with.

Now he is aware of the world beyond his mother, and for a time he is fearful of it and cannot cope. He therefore turns for safety to the person to whom he has become powerfully attached. Everyone else is for a time unwelcome.

This phase of 'stranger recognition' can be embarrassing and tiresome for the parents, but it is normal and necessary for good social and emotional development. It is a first step towards the child's ability to discriminate between strangers and those he loves, an ability to enter into enduring relationships in later life.

c. After about 9 months: Making Real Relationships

The fear of strangers lasts from two to eight weeks, during which time the baby may have withdrawn even from the father. But by eight to nine months he will turn to him again in a more mature way of relating. The strength of the baby's attachment to him reflects the extent of the father's availability and involvement. Father is known and enjoyed, but is as yet less important than the mother because his role as a breadwinner usually means that he has a smaller part in the ongoing care. But the father becomes increasingly important as the months and years go by.

Gradually the baby makes a few other relationships to close family members, and perhaps to family friends, but always according to the extent of their involvement with him. His behaviour towards people outside the family is reserved. He is now acutely aware of the difference between intimate family, friendly acquaintances, and strangers. The blood tie has no meaning for him. His relationship to a near neighbour may be closer than to a distant grandmother.

By the end of the first year the baby is crawling and perhaps walking, curious about the world around him; bravely moving a few yards away from the mother or father but speedily getting back to one of them as a place of safety if danger threatens, or if he is tired or hurt; friendly to familiar people outside the family but not indiscriminately so as when he was four or five months old.

d. After the first year

During the second and third years the importance of the child's attachment to his parents becomes clearer. In his relationship to them he begins to show 'giving' aspects of loving. He wants to share – even if it is only a corner of his sticky bun; he shows concern if he thinks a parent is hurt or unhappy, and wants to kiss them better.

He is beginning to love.

As he moves out of babyhood his parents begin to expect more grown-up behaviour, and because he loves them he tries to do what they ask of him. He is gradually expected to tolerate frustrations, to be toilet-trained, and to substitute language for impulsive action.

The child can accept these curbs because it is his parents who want this behaviour from him. He loves and wants to please them – wants to be in harmony with them, wants to be like them. The parents, because they are bonded to him, sympathize with the struggle within the child and give him time to comply; they are patient with backsliding, and give constant encouragement to his efforts.

At first he does what they ask of him only while they are there to remind him; but in time these codes of behaviour become his own and form the basis of his social behaviour outside the family.

What Happens to Bonding and Attachment?

There are many degrees of bonding, depending mainly upon the amount of the parents' involvement in the care of their child during the early years from birth. Some parents are unable to commit themselves deeply for personality reasons related to their own unsatisfactory childhood experiences; but in this book we are writing about the majority of ordinary parents who are capable of bonding fully to their children.

Parents who are bonded rarely act selfishly towards the child. His well-being takes priority, and whatever is in the child's interest feels right to them. They accept his love, tolerate his demands and failings, share his pain and pleasure – and get satisfaction from doing so. They may be sorely tried at times, but more than anyone else they are able to tolerate his growing pains.*

The child knows he is special to them, whether he is pleasing or not, well or ill, succeeding or failing. He unhesitatingly turns to them with his pleasures and miseries, confident that they will be there. He knows they are likely to see his point of view and give him the benefit of doubt before voicing critical comment.

They become the brick wall he can safely kick against. Impatient or angry though they may sometimes be, he recognizes that these are often signs of their concern for him.

His feelings about himself reflect his parents' feelings about him. The child whose parents value him values himself.

Parents usually carry these strong feelings throughout their lives – the love, the anxiety for their children's welfare and happiness. In a modified form these extend to their grandchildren. Bonding is a mature form of loving.

But the attachment of child to parents is an immature form of loving – unstable in the early months and years, with dependency as its main ingredient.

At adolescence, as the child achieves independence and moves towards adulthood, attachment to his parents lessens.

His feelings for his parents lose some of the earlier traits, and a caring attitude towards them eventually replaces the former dependency.

Having learned to love in his relationship with his parents, he marries and

---

*A 6-year-old: 'Your mother has to love you in case no one else does.'

A 7-year-old after having been out to tea: 'She's a funny mother. She's nicer to other people's children than her own.'

in due course bonds as deeply to his own children and becomes the object of their attachments.

So bonding progresses down the generations to promote the well-being of each new batch of babies.

Chapter Six

Conclusion

We have shown two babies, Paul and Sarah, who were mothered within the family throughout the first year, and it will be obvious that we consider this to be how a baby's emotional health and a family's relationships get the best start.

This is the choice of most parents. Like Katherine and Jean, the mother stays at home to tend the baby and finds pleasure and satisfaction in doing so.

But as with any other job that of caring for children brings with it at times tiredness, boredom and frustration. The mother loves and enjoys her baby, but when his activity requires constant vigilance to meet his needs and ensure his safety she can feel isolated and restricted.

To ease the constraints of the second year when toddlers are at their most demanding, many mothers take advantage of community facilities – mother–toddler clubs, one o'clock clubs, drop-in centres – where very young children play within reassuring reach of the mother; and where mothers meet with others similarly placed. These are valuable tension breakers.

Father, grandparents, and close friends – people the child knows and with whom he feels safe – can free the mother occasionally until such time as the child is ready for regular attendance at a playgroup.

Meeting the needs of young children throughout the first few years will bring its quota of difficulties; but for the parents there are exquisite rewards, and for the child good experiences that will affect his whole life.

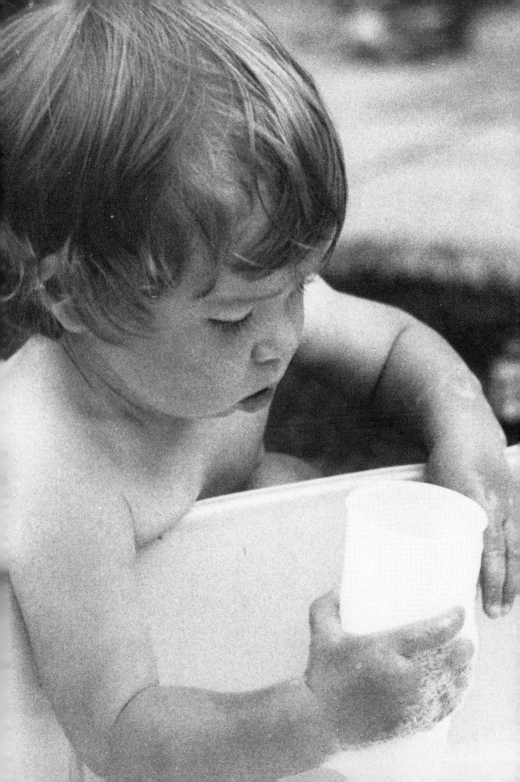

References

1. D.W. Winnicott, 'Getting to Know Your Baby', in *The Child, the Family and the Outside World*, Pelican Books, 1964.
2. M.K. Klaus and J.H. Kennell, *Maternal-Infant Bonding*, C.V. Mosby, St Louis, U.S.A., 1976.
3. H. Nagera, 'Day Care Centres: Red Light, Green Light, or Amber Light?', *Int. Rev. Psychoanal.*, vol. 1, 1974, pp. 137–71.
4. J.C. Spence, *The Purpose of the Family: A Guide to the Care of Children*, Epworth Press, 1946.
5. Klaus and Kennell, op. cit.
6. Health Services Commissioner (Ombudsman), *Selected Investigations Completed 1979–1980, 4th Report*, H.M.S.O., 1980, pp. 149–55.
7. National Association for the Welfare of Children in Hospital, Exton House, 7 Exton Street, London, SE1 (01-261 1738).

American Association for the Care of Children in Hospital, 3625 Wisconsin Avenue, Washington D.C. 20016, U.S.A. (202-244 1801).

Australian Association for the Welfare of Children in Hospital, 78 Phillip Street, Parramatta, N.S.W. 2150, Australia (635 4785).
8. James Robertson, *Young Children in Hospital*, Tavistock, 1977 (Third Edition).
9. Ministry of Health (Central Health Services Council), *The Welfare of Children in Hospital: Report of the Committee* (The Platt Report), H.M.S.O., 1959.
10. Joyce Robertson, 'Mothering as an Influence on Early Development. A Study of Well Baby Clinic Records', *Psychoanal. Study Child*, no. 17, 1962, pp. 245–64.
11. J. and J. Robertson, 'The Psychological Parent', *Adoption and Fostering*, no. 1, 1977, pp. 19–22.

FILMS BY JAMES AND JOYCE ROBERTSON

(16mm, sound. There are Danish, French, German and Swedish versions of some of the films.)

A Two-Year-Old Goes to Hospital
Going to Hospital with Mother
John, *17 months, for 9 days in a residential nursery*
Jane, *17 months, in foster care for 10 days*
Lucy, *21 months, in foster care for 21 days*
Thomas, *2 years 4 months, in foster care for 10 days*
Kate, *2 years 5 months, in foster care*

'The demonstrations *ad oculos* offered by these films are to my mind direct observation at its best' – Anna Freud

'... as good as a textbook on children's emotional needs. Each film is a miniature work of art. Not to know them is to miss a rare treat. Indispensable for child study classes and for all who deal with very young children' – *Audiovisuals for Mental Health Education*, 1979

Available from

Concord Films Council, Ipswich, Suffolk, England
New York University Film Library, U.S.A.